Journey to Inception of Life

Troubleshooting in ART Laboratory

Journey to Inception of Life

Troubleshooting in ART Laboratory

Editors

Chandan Vijay Salunke PhD
Clinical Embryologist
Managing Director
Kasturi ReproAssist Concepts LLP
Panjim, Goa, India

Shravani Kanakdas Parker MSc
Clinical Embryologist
Executive Director
Kasturi ReproAssist Concepts LLP
Panjim, Goa, India

Foreword

Ameet A Naik

JAYPEE

JAYPEE BROTHERS MEDICAL PUBLISHERS
The Health Sciences Publisher
New Delhi | London

Jaypee Brothers Medical Publishers (P) Ltd

Headquarters
EMCA House, 23/23-B
Ansari Road, Daryaganj
New Delhi 110 002, India
Landline: +91-11-23272143, +91-11-23272703
+91-11-23282021, +91-11-23245672
e-mail: jaypee@jaypeebrothers.com

Corporate Office
4838/24, Ansari Road, Daryaganj
New Delhi 110 002, India
Phone: +91-11-43574357
Fax: +91-11-43574314
e-mail: jaypee@jaypeebrothers.com

Overseas Office
JP Medical Ltd
83 Victoria Street, London
SW1H 0HW (UK)
Phone: +44-20 3170 8910
e-mail: info@jpmedpub.com

EU GPSR Authorised Representative
Logos Europe, 9 rue Nicolas Poussin
17000, La Rochelle, France
Phone: +33 (0) 6 67 93 73 78
e-mail: contact@logoseurope.eu

Website: www.jaypeebrothers.com
Website: www.jaypeedigital.com

Journey to Inception of Life: Troubleshooting in ART Laboratory

First Edition: **2026**

ISBN: 978-93-7202-526-2

Printed at: Samrat Offset Pvt. Ltd.

Dedication

To our dearest parents

You stood silently behind our every milestone, offering wisdom

when we faltered and patience when we doubted.

Your values of humility, discipline, and compassion

became the unseen scaffolding of this work.

This book may carry our names,

but its roots are firmly planted in your unwavering love.

May these pages honor the sacrifices

you never spoke of, but we never forgot.

Foreword

In the landscape of modern reproductive medicine, precision is no longer a luxury, it is a necessity. Every step in the assisted reproductive technology (ART) laboratory, from gamete handling to embryo transfer, holds the weight of human dreams. Yet, behind the apparent standardization of procedures lies a lesser addressed reality: troubleshooting.

Journey to Inception of Life: Troubleshooting in ART Laboratory, authored by Dr Chandan Vijay Salunke and Ms Shravani Kanakdas Parker, arrives at a crucial juncture in ART practice. As a clinician, I have seen firsthand how outcomes can hinge not just on the protocols followed, but on the ability of the embryologist to navigate the unexpected, to identify anomalies, to rectify deviations, and to adapt quickly with both scientific rigor and clinical intuition.

This book acknowledges the unpredictable terrain that every embryologist, and by extension every ART team, must learn to traverse. What makes this work exceptional is its fusion of scientific clarity with real-world laboratory insights. The authors bring together years of experience, countless observations, and a shared passion for precision to craft a volume that serves as both reference and reflection.

It is not just a guide for when things go wrong, it is a manual to help us to understand *why* they go wrong, *how* to interpret the signs, and *what* can be done to restore balance in the culture system, equipment calibration, gamete quality, or even human error pathways. Their work builds a bridge between embryology theory and clinical practice, one that every ART professional should cross.

Moreover, the book represents something rare: An honest, methodical, and deeply human approach to improving patient's outcomes. It recognizes that behind every dish, every drop of media, and every manipulated gamete, there lies not only a scientific challenge but also an ethical responsibility.

May this become more than a manual, may it become a movement toward better practices, fewer errors, and ultimately more fulfilled dreams.

Ameet A Naik
MBBS MD (Obs & Gyne)
Fellow of Endoscopic Surgery
Diploma in Reproductive Medicine
Director
Platicare Hospital and Platicare IVF
Ponda, Goa, India

Preface

Assisted reproductive technology (ART) stands at the confluence of precise science and profound human emotion. It is a domain where microscopic decisions carry macroscopic consequences, where a shift in pH, a deviation in temperature, or a single overlooked parameter can silently alter the trajectory of life itself. In this space of extraordinary delicacy, troubleshooting is not just a technical intervention; it is a clinical imperative.

This book was born out of lived experiences within the embryology laboratory, a place that is as much about protocols as it is about patience, as much about results as it is about responsibility. Through the years, we found that while training programs and textbooks teach procedures, far fewer resources truly address the *why* behind failures or the *how* to intervene when things deviate from ideal. This gap, often encountered in the silence after a failed fertilization, a sudden embryo arrest, or an unexplained thawing outcome, called for a structured, evidence-based, and context-aware compilation of practical knowledge. This book is our response.

Journey to Inception of Life: Troubleshooting in ART Laboratory is designed not as a protocol manual, but as a *scientific companion* also to those who seek to understand the subtleties behind common pitfalls in ART. It brings together research, real-world case reflections, and the evolving best practices that have helped to shape more resilient, reproducible, and ethical embryology practices.

The structure of the book follows the natural timeline of an IVF cycle; from semen processing and oocyte handling to fertilization, embryo culture, cryopreservation, and embryo transfer, for each step, we explore the critical points where errors may arise. Every chapter is laced with both biological rationale and technical resolution, keeping in mind the rigors of international standards and the emotional realities of patients and practitioners alike.

Our hope is that this book will not only enhance your technical understanding but also deepen your respect for the fragile and miraculous path from gamete to embryo to life.

We invite you to walk this journey with scientific rigor, ethical clarity, and a continued curiosity for in every embryo lies a story waiting to be told, and in every challenge, an opportunity to learn.

Chandan Vijay Salunke
Shravani Kanakdas Parker

Acknowledgments

This book is the culmination of many years spent immersed in the intricate world of "Assisted Reproductive Technology (ART)" that brings together the precision of science with the quiet strength of human hope. The pages that follow are not just techniques and troubleshooting protocols; they are reflections of real challenges faced, problems solved, and lives transformed; including our own.

We are deeply grateful to the patients and couples whose silent stories form the invisible thread connecting every case, every laboratory decision, and every meaningful outcome. Their resilience has shaped our sense of purpose as professionals in this field.

To the mentors, colleagues, and peers in reproductive science, thank you for fostering critical thinking, upholding scientific integrity and sharing your curiosity. Your insights, feedback, and constant pursuit of improvement have guided our growth and strengthened this work.

We acknowledge the many institutions, IVF laboratories and scientific communities that offered us their resources, data, and spaces for learning. This book carries forward the cumulative wisdom we gained through those experiences.

To our families and friends, your constant encouragement, quiet patience, and belief in our journey allowed us to pursue this demanding work with clarity and conviction. Your support has been the quiet foundation beneath everything we have built.

And to the readers, aspiring embryologists, researchers, and clinicians, who take up the complex yet rewarding path of ART; we hope this book supports your practice with clarity, humility, and the shared goal of making life possible, one cell at a time.

Chandan Vijay Salunke
Shravani Kanakdas Parker

Contents

SECTION 1

Foundations of Troubleshooting in Assisted Reproductive Technology

CHAPTER 1

Introduction to Troubleshooting in Assisted Reproductive Technology

OVERVIEW AND SIGNIFICANCE

Assisted reproductive technology (ART) has evolved from an experimental medical intervention to a highly specialized and regulated domain of reproductive science. Since the birth of Louise Brown in 1978, the world's first baby conceived via in-vitro fertilization (IVF), ART has undergone exponential growth in its scope, reliability, and complexity.[1-8] From basic IVF and intracytoplasmic sperm injection (ICSI) to preimplantation genetic testing and embryo vitrification, ART procedures are now performed across a wide range of indications. While technological advancements and refined protocols have improved success rates, the sensitivity of human gametes and embryos to environmental, procedural, and biochemical changes still demands vigilant observation **(Fig. 1)**. These require timely corrective action; commonly referred to as "troubleshooting."

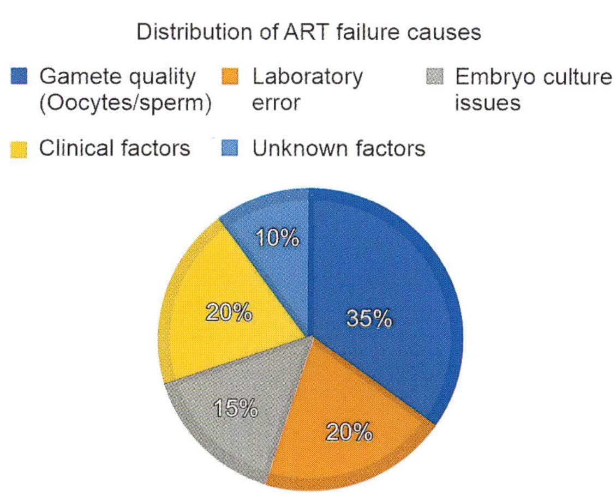

Fig. 1: Data derived from published assisted reproductive technology (ART) failure audits, 2010–2020.

Troubleshooting is not merely reactive; it is a structured, evidence-based process that forms a foundational pillar of ART quality control. It involves the identification, evaluation, and resolution of deviations, nonconformities, and potential errors across the laboratory workflow from gamete retrieval and handling to embryo culture, cryopreservation, and transfer.[6]

HISTORICAL EVOLUTION OF TROUBLESHOOTING IN ASSISTED REPRODUCTIVE TECHNOLOGY

In the early years of IVF, laboratory troubleshooting relied heavily on the intuition and observational skills of embryologists. Limited instrumentation, variable culture systems, and inconsistencies in media preparation made early ART cycles unpredictable. Common problems such as poor embryo cleavage, oocyte degeneration, or low fertilization were often attributed to "bad luck" or patient's variability rather than process failure.[3]

With the introduction of sequential culture media,[4] time-lapse embryo imaging, and micromanipulation systems like ICSI,[4] embryologists were granted unprecedented insight into gamete and embryo behavior **(Table 1)**. This transition necessitated a shift toward proactive troubleshooting, where pattern recognition, root-cause analysis, and corrective action plans became essential.[2] Over time, global standards, including ISO 15189 for laboratory accreditation, European Society of Human Reproduction and Embryology (ESHRE) guidelines for IVF laboratories, and local

TABLE 1: Key milestones in the evolution of assisted reproductive technology (ART) and laboratory practices.

Year	Milestone	Description
1978	First IVF baby (Louise Brown, UK)	Birth of the first baby via in-vitro fertilization (IVF)
1983	First pregnancy via donor egg IVF	Expansion of IVF using donor gametes
1984	First frozen embryo transfer (FET)	Use of cryopreserved embryos
1986	Birth of first baby from cryopreserved embryo	Proof of concept for embryo freezing
1992	Introduction of ICSI (Palermo et al.)	Revolution in male infertility treatment via direct sperm injection
1995	Blastocyst culture and transfer	Improved implantation rates using day 5 embryos
1999	Vitrification techniques developed	Rapid freezing, better survival of oocytes/embryos
2001	Clinical PGT for aneuploidy and disease	Genetic testing before embryo transfer
2010	Time-lapse embryo imaging	Real-time monitoring for better embryo selection
2012	Oocyte vitrification recognized as standard	Elective egg freezing and fertility preservation
2015	*CRISPR* gene editing in embryos (Experimental)	Ethical debates on embryo gene editing begin
2020	AI-based embryo selection introduced	Noninvasive and automated embryo grading

regulations like the ART Act (India, 2021), have formalized troubleshooting as a non-negotiable component of laboratory competence.

SCOPE OF TROUBLESHOOTING IN ASSISTED REPRODUCTIVE TECHNOLOGY

Troubleshooting in ART is an interdisciplinary effort that spans equipment, media, personnel, documentation, and clinical interface. Each ART procedure comprises 100s of micro-steps, where even slight deviations—like a 0.5°C temperature drop or exposure to VOCs, can result in irreversible biological damage. Common areas include:

Equipment and Infrastructure

Malfunctioning CO_2 incubators, uncalibrated micropipettes, incorrect micromanipulator axis alignment, or failure of high-efficiency particulate air (HEPA) filtration.

Consumables and Reagents

Lot-to-lot media variability, expired oil overlay, defective culture dishes, endotoxin contamination, or residual detergent in wash buffers.[2]

Gamete and Embryo Handling

Shearing stress during pipetting, overexposure to hyaluronidase, incorrect temperature during ICSI, or oocyte lysis during denudation.[7]

Environmental Factors

Volatile organic compounds (VOCs), improper humidity, airflow disturbances, light exposure, or condensate in dish lids.[9,10]

Documentation and Traceability

Sample mislabeling, missing logs for cryostorage, absence of witnessing, or incomplete consent forms—potentially leading to legal consequences.

Regulatory and Ethical Noncompliance

Assisted reproductive technology Act violations, improper gamete sourcing, failure in record retention, or nonconformity with surrogacy regulations.

PRINCIPLES OF EFFECTIVE TROUBLESHOOTING

Root Cause Analysis

Effective troubleshooting relies on identifying not just what went wrong, but why. Root cause analysis (RCA) methodologies, such as the Fishbone (Ishikawa) diagram, which help to dissect problems into categories: equipment, environment, technique, human error, or systemic fault.

Corrective and Preventive Actions

A vital component of ART laboratory quality systems, corrective and preventive actions (CAPA) ensures that identified problems are rectified (corrective) and future occurrences are prevented (preventive), as outlined in ISO 9001:2015 and ESHRE's Key Performance Indicators for ART laboratories[1] **(Flowchart 1)**.

Real-time Monitoring and Trend Analysis

Tracking nonconformities over time—such as frequent embryo arrest at the 8-cell stage—can uncover subtle systemic issues like media degradation or faulty gas mixtures.

Training and Competency

Untrained personnel or inconsistent execution of protocols can lead to recurring errors. Regular competency assessments, SOP reviews, and mentorship play critical roles in fostering a troubleshooting culture.[5] To ensure standardized operations, SOPs should clearly delineate the responsibilities assigned to senior, junior, and trainee embryologists. Rotational sharing of maintenance tasks and procedural duties promotes accountability and reduces error redundancy. Periodic re-evaluation and updates of SOPs also accommodate advances in equipment, techniques, and regulatory expectations, ensuring relevance and compliance across all levels of personnel.

Flowchart 1: *Troubleshooting workflow:* Root cause analysis and corrective and preventive actions (CAPA) in assisted reproductive technology (ART) laboratories.

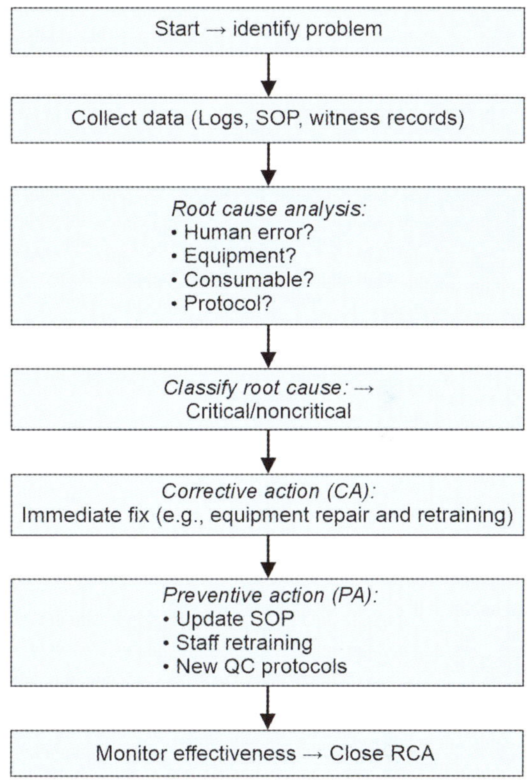

GLOBAL FRAMEWORKS AND GUIDELINES SUPPORTING TROUBLESHOOTING

International agencies have established detailed recommendations to guide troubleshooting protocols **(Table 2)**.

ROLE OF THE EMBRYOLOGIST IN TROUBLESHOOTING

An embryologist is not merely a technician but a biological detective. Identifying a subtle change in pronuclear appearance, cytoplasmic granularity, or delayed compaction can alert the team to errors in pH, osmolality, or temperature that may not be apparent on routine checks. Embryologists must function as sentinels of

TABLE 2: Key regulatory and quality standards relevant to troubleshooting in assisted reproductive technology (ART) laboratories.

Organization	*Guideline/standard*	*Relevance*
ESHRE	Guidelines on Laboratory Setup, Witnessing, and KPIs (2022)	Troubleshooting linked to performance metrics, media use, and embryo grading
WHO	Laboratory Manual for the Examination of Human Semen (6th Edition)	Semen analysis and processing errors
ICMR (India)	ART (Regulation) Act, 2021	Legal compliance, donor handling, traceability, and cryopreservation logs
ISO	ISO 14644 (Cleanrooms), ISO 15189 (Laboratory Quality), ISO 20387 (Biobanking)	Infrastructure, calibration, and cryostorage errors

Note: By aligning troubleshooting practices with these frameworks, ART centers improve both clinical outcomes and compliance with legal/ethical expectations.
(ESHRE: European Society of Human Reproduction and Embryology; ICMR: Indian Council of Medical Research; KPIs: key performance indicators; WHO: World Health Organization)

biological quality—documenting, analyzing, and reporting deviations with clarity and objectivity.[9]

Troubleshooting also demands psychological resilience. ART cycles are emotionally charged, and embryologists carry the burden of decisions that can determine the fate of a patient's reproductive effort. A culture of open communication, nonpunitive error reporting, and continual learning is essential to sustain performance under pressure.

TOWARD A CULTURE OF TROUBLESHOOTING IN ASSISTED REPRODUCTIVE TECHNOLOGY

To institutionalize troubleshooting in ART laboratories, the following practices are recommended:

- *Daily huddles:* Brief morning reviews of equipment status, ongoing cases, and unusual findings.
- *Deviation logs:* Structured recording of all nonconformities with follow-up and closure.
- *Simulations and drills:* Regular response protocols for incidents such as power failure, LN_2 spill, or mislabeling events.
- *Digitalization:* Integration of Laboratory Information Management Systems (LIMS), environmental monitors, and e-witnessing for traceability.
- *Audit Trails and CAPA Boards:* Visual tracking of open issues and CAPA implementation deadlines.

These elements contribute to a laboratory ecosystem that is resilient, transparent, and geared toward continuous improvement.

CONCLUSION

Troubleshooting in ART is more than a response to failure—it is a proactive and systemic safeguard that bridges science, ethics, and patient care. By recognizing subtle patterns, engaging in structured analysis, and aligning with global standards, ART professionals can protect biological integrity, prevent cycle failure, and uphold trust in reproductive care. As reproductive science continues to evolve, the ability to troubleshoot effectively will remain the hallmark of a competent and compassionate ART laboratory.

REFERENCES

1. Alpha Scientists in Reproductive Medicine and ESHRE Special Interest Group of Embryology. The Vienna Consensus: Recommended performance indicators for clinical and laboratory assisted reproductive technology. Hum Reprod Open. 2011;2011(1):1-19.
2. ESHRE Guideline Group on Good Practice in IVF Labs; De los Santos MJ, Apter S, Coticchio G, Debrock S, Lundin K, et al. Revised guidelines for good practice in IVF laboratories. Hum Reprod. 2016;31(4):685-6.
3. Edwards RG, Purdy JM. Human conception in vitro. Hum Reprod. 1982;3(1):51-62.
4. Gardner DK, Lane M. Culture and selection of viable blastocysts: A viable strategy for transfer. J Assist Reprod Genet. 1993;10(10):558-63.
5. Maher J, Meniru G. Troubleshooting in IVF: A Laboratory Guide. New York: Informa Healthcare; 2005.
6. Morbeck DE, Leonard PH, Hill MJ. Disparate impact of oil overlay on human embryo development and media osmolality. J Assist Reprod Genet. 2017;34(6):733-9.
7. Palermo G, Joris H, Devroey P, Van Steirteghem AC. Pregnancies after intracytoplasmic injection of single spermatozoon into an oocyte. Lancet. 1992;340(8810):17-8.
8. Steptoe PC, Edwards RG. Birth after the reimplantation of a human embryo. Lancet. 1978;2(8085):366.
9. Swain JE. Optimizing the culture environment in the IVF laboratory: Impact of pH and buffer capacity on gamete and embryo quality. Reprod Biomed Online. 2012;24(5):484-90.
10. Swain JE, Pool TB. ART failure: development of an assay to detect embryo toxicity in IVF culture media. Reprod Biomed Online. 2008;16(3):401-8.

SECTION

2 Gamete Analysis and Preparation

CHAPTER 2 Quality Control in Assisted Reproductive Technology Laboratory

INTRODUCTION

Quality control (QC) in assisted reproductive technology (ART) laboratories is a fundamental aspect of maintaining the safety, consistency, and reliability of clinical outcomes. The process of fertilization and embryo development is highly sensitive to external factors, and any variation in laboratory conditions can adversely affect the viability and quality of gametes and embryos. For instance, fluctuations in carbon dioxide (CO_2) levels may alter the pH of culture media, potentially impairing embryo cleavage or arresting development. Exposure to volatile organic compounds such as alcohols or aromatic chemicals from cleaning agents or laboratory materials can disrupt zona pellucida integrity and decrease blastocyst expansion potential. Similarly, airborne particles from cotton-based clothing, improperly maintained filters, or substandard airflow systems may introduce contaminants that lead to higher rates of fragmentation or developmental failure. These issues are often avoidable with the implementation of stringent QC protocols. A comprehensive QC framework involves continuous monitoring of air quality, temperature, humidity, gas concentrations, and sterility levels through calibrated equipment and validated processes. The use of cleanroom infrastructure, including lint-free laboratory garments, high-efficiency particulate air (HEPA) filters, epoxy-coated floors, and digitally controlled incubators, further supports an optimal microenvironment for embryo culture. Regular swab testing, volatile organic compounds (VOCs) level assessments, oxygen depletion monitoring, and environmental mapping are integral to contamination prevention. Adherence to established international standards, such as ISO 14644 for airborne cleanliness, ISO 17025 for equipment calibration, and ESHRE guidelines for ART laboratory setup and practice, ensures that laboratory environments remain consistent and compliant with the best practices in reproductive medicine. Therefore, QC is not simply a technical requirement but a critical component of clinical success and patient's safety in ART programs.

AIR QUALITY MANAGEMENT AND VOLATILE ORGANIC COMPOUNDS CONTROL

Air quality in ART laboratories is a critical determinant of embryological and clinical success, as airborne particulates, VOCs, and microbial contaminants can interfere with the delicate physiology of gametes and embryos. These contaminants may originate from external environments, human activity, heating, ventilation, and air conditioning (HVAC) systems, equipment off-gassing, or even consumables. To mitigate these risks, ART laboratories are designed with advanced air handling systems incorporating HEPA filters for removal of particles down to 0.3 μ, and activated carbon filters that adsorb VOCs such as formaldehyde, plasticizers, and solvents. Positive pressure airflow is used to prevent ingress of unfiltered air into sensitive laboratory zones. In addition to centralized filtration systems, the installation of standalone air purifiers equipped with both HEPA and activated carbon modules is increasingly recommended, particularly in zones with high personnel activity or consumable unpacking. It is crucial, however, that laboratories avoid the use of ultraviolet (UV) light or chemical fumigation, which can degrade plastics and generate secondary VOCs harmful to embryos. Instead, regular filter and prefilter maintenance protocols must be followed, including scheduled replacement based on particle load monitoring. Prefilters, which trap coarse particulates before air reaches the HEPA unit, play a vital role in extending the lifespan and efficiency of primary filters and should not be overlooked. Maintaining a sterile, particle-controlled, and VOC-free atmosphere through these combined strategies is essential to ensure optimal culture conditions and to minimize embryo stress during critical windows of development **(Table 1)**.

TABLE 1: Air quality parameters and their impact.

Parameter	*Description*	*Impact on ART outcomes*	*Solution*
Particulate matter (PM)	PM includes dust, aerosols, and other fine particles that can introduce contaminants and disrupt air cleanliness. Particulates can adhere to laboratory surfaces or culture media, introducing physical and chemical contaminants that affect gamete and embryo health	High PM levels increase contamination risks, reduce embryo viability, and alter gamete and embryo metabolism. PMs can carry VOCs and microbial contaminants that increase oxidative stress, disrupt cell membrane integrity, and hinder zygote and embryo development[3]	Use HEPA filters with an efficiency of 99.97% to remove particulates as small as 0.3 μ. Regularly replace and validate HEPA filters to maintain efficiency. Implement laminar airflow systems and positive pressure setups to prevent unfiltered air from entering the laboratory[4]
Volatile organic compounds (VOCs)	VOCs are organic chemicals that easily evaporate and become airborne. Sources include construction materials, laboratory equipment, cleaning agents, and consumables. Common VOCs include formaldehyde, benzene, and xylene, which are known to be cytotoxic and disrupt cellular function	VOCs contribute to oxidative stress, increased ROS levels, and cellular damage. They disrupt DNA integrity and protein synthesis, leading to reduced fertilization and embryo fragmentation. VOCs can induce mitochondrial dysfunction, impaired ATP production, and increased apoptosis[1]	Use activated carbon filters to adsorb VOCs and gaseous contaminants. Avoid using VOC-emitting materials and replace them with VOC-free alternatives. Regularly monitor VOC levels using real-time VOC detectors or gas chromatography. Implement ventilation systems with high air exchange rates to dilute VOC concentrations. Avoid use of perfumes, colorants, and alcohol-based agents such as spirit or sanitizer in or near laboratory areas. Ensure that wall and surface coatings are VOC-free and that materials are compliant with low-emission standards[2]

Contd...

Contd...

Parameter	*Description*	*Impact on ART outcomes*	*Solution*
Total volatile organic compounds (TVOCs)	TVOCs represent the cumulative concentration of all VOCs present in the air. High TVOC levels indicate overall poor air quality and increased cytotoxicity risks. TVOCs are measured in micrograms per cubic meter ($\mu g/m^3$) and should be kept as low as possible	Elevated TVOCs are linked to poor embryo development, increased apoptosis, and higher rates of embryo degeneration. Prolonged exposure can result in persistent oxidative stress and long-term reproductive failure. TVOC levels above 50 $\mu g/m^3$ are considered unsafe for ART laboratory environments[3]	Regularly monitor TVOC levels using portable meters or fixed VOC monitoring systems. Use oil overlays on culture dishes to minimize the direct exposure of gametes and embryos to ambient air. Maintain TVOC levels below 20 $\mu g/m^3$, as recommended by ESHRE guidelines. Implement air quality control plans with periodic audits to detect and rectify TVOC sources[2]
Microbial contaminants	Airborne bacteria, fungi, and spores can contaminate culture media and equipment, leading to infections and disrupted gamete and embryo development. Sources include personnel, HVAC systems, and open dish exposure. Airborne contaminants can introduce endotoxins that impair embryo development and cause immunogenic responses	Microbial contamination leads to poor-quality embryos, reduced fertilization rates, and increased incidence of embryonic degeneration. Bacterial endotoxins can disrupt cellular signaling, induce inflammatory responses, and alter gene expression, resulting in failed embryo development[2]	Implement positive pressure air systems with HEPA filtration to limit microbial entry. Use air sampling assays, such as settle plates and air samplers, to monitor microbial load. Apply regular disinfection protocols and UV sterilization of workstations and incubators. Validate cleanroom environments according to ISO 14698 standards[4]

AIR HANDLING SYSTEMS AND FILTRATION TECHNOLOGIES

- *High-efficiency particulate air and ultra-low penetration air (ULPA) filters:* HEPA and ULPA filters are designed to remove particulates as small as 0.1 µ with an efficiency of 99.99%. These filters prevent the circulation of contaminants, ensuring a cleanroom environment. Regular replacement and validation are required to maintain filter efficiency.
- *Activated carbon filters:* Activated carbon filters adsorb VOCs and other gaseous contaminants, effectively reducing cytotoxic agents in the laboratory air. When combined with HEPA filters, they enhance air quality by capturing both particulate and volatile contaminants. Monitor filter performance using breakthrough indicators or VOC meters.
- *Air exchange and positive pressure systems:* Positive pressure systems prevent the entry of unfiltered air into the cleanroom, reducing contamination risks. An air exchange rate of 15–20 changes per hour is recommended to maintain cleanroom conditions and dilute airborne contaminants effectively. Regular validation and maintenance of air handling units are essential.

- *Environmental monitoring systems:* Use real-time monitoring systems to track air quality parameters, including particulate count, VOC concentration, CO_2 levels, and microbial load. Implement automated alerts for parameter deviations to enable prompt corrective actions.

TEMPERATURE AND HUMIDITY CONTROL

Temperature and humidity control are crucial for maintaining the stability of culture media and the viability of gametes and embryos. Fluctuations in temperature or humidity can cause thermal shock, alter osmolarity, and impair cellular function, resulting in developmental anomalies or compromised embryo quality. The use of dehumidifiers helps to maintain consistent humidity levels, especially in tropical or monsoon climates, preventing condensation and microbial growth within the laboratory environment.

TEMPERATURE REGULATION

Temperature stability is vital for preventing thermal shock and maintaining cellular homeostasis **(Table 2)**. Ideal room temperatures should be between 22 and 25°C, while incubators, workstations, and culture media should be maintained at 37°C. Fluctuations in temperature can lead to altered enzyme activity, disrupted protein synthesis, and impaired embryo development.

HUMIDITY REGULATION

Humidity levels in ART laboratories should be maintained between 40 and 60%. Low humidity increases evaporation rates, altering osmolarity and pH of culture media, while high humidity can cause condensation, promoting microbial growth and contamination **(Table 3)**.

TABLE 2: Troubleshooting temperature-related errors in assisted reproductive technology (ART) laboratories.

Issue	*Description*	*Impact on ART outcomes*	*Solution*
Temperature fluctuations	Sudden changes in temperature can result from HVAC malfunctions, frequent opening of incubators, or prolonged dish exposure. Even brief temperature drops can affect cellular function and embryo metabolism	Temperature variations impact cellular processes, leading to altered gene expression, impaired mitochondrial function, and reduced blastocyst formation rates. Severe fluctuations can induce cell death or developmental arrest[2]	Use temperature-controlled incubators and workstations to maintain a constant 37°C. Monitor temperature in real-time using calibrated thermocouples and data loggers. Implement double door systems and minimize opening times to reduce temperature fluctuations. Regularly calibrate temperature sensors as per ISO/IEC 17025 standards[1]
Suboptimal temperature of culture media	Temperature deviations in culture media can result from inadequate equilibration, prolonged handling times, or faulty heating systems	Suboptimal temperatures affect cellular metabolism, disrupt cytoskeletal integrity, and compromise developmental potential. Incorrect media temperature can lead to failed fertilization or abnormal embryo development[2]	Ensure that all culture media and solutions are preequilibrated to 37°C before use. Minimize dish exposure times and use temperature-controlled stages for micromanipulation procedures. Monitor media temperatures using temperature probes and data loggers to ensure consistency. Implement preventive maintenance and regular calibration of heating system[1]

(HVAC: heating, ventilation, and air conditioning)

TABLE 3: Troubleshooting humidity-related issues in assisted reproductive technology (ART) laboratories.

Issue	*Description*	*Impact on ART outcomes*	*Solution*
Low humidity and increased evaporation	Low humidity leads to increased evaporation of culture media, resulting in altered osmolarity and pH. This can cause osmotic stress on gametes and embryos, affecting cellular viability and function	Low humidity and increased evaporation lead to osmotic imbalance, impaired membrane function, and reduced fertilization rates. Altered osmolarity can cause cell shrinkage or swelling, impacting embryo viability[3]	Use humidification systems within incubators to maintain stable humidity. Seal culture dishes with oil overlays to reduce evaporation. Monitor humidity levels using calibrated hygrometers and implement automated humidity control systems in culture rooms and incubators
High humidity and condensation	High humidity levels promote condensation within incubators and culture dishes, increasing the risk of microbial contamination and disrupting the microenvironment of gametes and embryos	High humidity levels lead to microbial growth, increased contamination risks, and potential chemical interactions within culture media. Condensation alters gas exchange and can cause localized shifts in pH and osmolarity[3]	Use dehumidifiers in culture rooms and maintain air circulation to prevent condensation. Implement regular cleaning and sterilization protocols for incubators and culture rooms. Ensure that incubators are equipped with humidity sensors and perform regular maintenance and calibration[4]

CONTAMINATION PREVENTION AND MONITORING ASSAYS

Contamination in ART laboratories can arise from a variety of sources, including personnel, equipment, and consumables. Contaminants such as bacteria, fungi, and chemical residues can compromise embryo quality, leading to failed fertilization or implantation. Implementing rigorous contamination prevention and monitoring strategies is essential for maintaining a sterile environment **(Table 4)**.

CONTAMINATION MONITORING ASSAYS

- *Settle plates and air samplers:* Settle plates are placed in critical areas to monitor microbial contamination over time. Air samplers actively capture air samples onto culture media, providing quantitative data on microbial load.
- *Surface swabbing and contact plates:* Surface swabs and contact plates are used to assess the cleanliness of work surfaces, equipment, and personnel gowns. These assays are critical for detecting bacterial or fungal contamination and validating cleaning protocols.
- *Chemical residue testing:* Chemical residues, such as detergents or disinfectants, can be cytotoxic to gametes and embryos. Regular testing for chemical residues using gas chromatography or liquid chromatography-mass spectrometry (LC-MS) is recommended to ensure no toxic residues remain on equipment or surfaces.

IMPLEMENTING A COMPREHENSIVE QUALITY CONTROL PROGRAM

A comprehensive QC program in ART laboratories involves the integration of various monitoring and validation techniques to maintain a stable and sterile environment. The program should

TABLE 4: Sources of contamination in assisted reproductive technology (ART) laboratories and troubleshooting measures.

Source of contamination	*Description*	*Impact on ART outcomes*	*Solution*
Personnel	Personnel are a major source of contamination, introducing microbial contaminants through skin, hair, and clothing. Human activities increase particulate and microbial load in the air	Increased microbial load and VOCs from personnel lead to higher contamination risks, reduced embryo quality, and lower success rates in ART	Implement strict gowning and personal hygiene protocols. Use gloves, masks, and sterile clothing. Monitor personnel behavior to minimize unnecessary movement in critical areas. Perform regular air and surface sampling of all working platforms to assess contamination levels[4]
Equipment and consumables	Equipment, pipettes, and consumables can introduce contaminants if not properly sterilized. Open dish exposure during handling can also increase contamination risks	Contaminated equipment leads to direct contact contamination, resulting in failed fertilization or embryo degeneration	Use sterile, single-use consumables whenever possible. Implement rigorous cleaning and autoclaving protocols for reusable equipment. Validate sterility using microbiological assays or endotoxin tests. Consider γ-irradiation for sterilization of critical consumables[2]
Surface and airborne contaminants	Surface contamination from dust, VOCs, or microbial growth can transfer to culture media, affecting embryo development. Airborne contaminants include particulates, aerosols, and VOCs	Contaminated surfaces or air leads to failed fertilization, embryo fragmentation, and developmental arrest	Implement strict surface cleaning protocols using nontoxic disinfectants. Use UV sterilization and HEPA-filtered airflow systems to minimize airborne contaminants. Monitor contamination using settle plates, contact plates, and air samplers. Regularly perform environmental microbial assays[1]

(HEPA: high-efficiency particulate air; UV: ultraviolet; VOCs: volatile organic compounds)

include regular environmental monitoring, validation of equipment and consumables, and adherence to international standards such as ISO 14644 for cleanroom classification and ISO 20387 for laboratory calibration.

- *Regular environmental monitoring:* Implement continuous monitoring of air quality, temperature, humidity, and contamination using real-time sensors and assays. Conduct weekly and monthly validation checks to ensure compliance with established standards.
- *Validation and calibration of equipment:* Perform regular calibration of critical equipment such as incubators, laminar airflow hoods, and VOC filters according to ISO/IEC 17025 standards. Use certified reference materials and follow strict protocols for calibration.
- *Staff training and compliance:* Regularly train staff on QC protocols, contamination prevention, and equipment handling. Implement competency assessments and refresher training sessions to ensure adherence to QC measures.

- *Documentation and auditing:* Maintain detailed records of all QC activities, including environmental monitoring, equipment validation, and contamination assays. Conduct internal and external audits to identify areas for improvement and ensure compliance with international standards.

CONCLUSION

Quality control in ART laboratories is not a static checklist, but a continuous cycle of vigilance, validation, and refinement. From air quality and media performance to equipment calibration and personnel competence, each element contributes to the delicate balance required for successful fertilization and embryo development. Even minor lapses such as unnoticed VOCs, unvalidated media lots, or improper storage can significantly compromise outcomes. A robust QC system ensures reproducibility, reduces variability, and builds trust with both patients and regulatory authorities. As ART continues to advance, the emphasis must shift from reactive troubleshooting to proactive quality assurance, with documentation, traceability, and outcome monitoring forming the foundation of a truly reliable laboratory ecosystem.

REFERENCES

1. Esfandiari N, Nazemian Z. Impact of volatile organic compounds on in vitro fertilization and embryo development. J Assist Reprod Genet. 2017;34(10):1345-54.
2. Gardner DK, Kelley RL. Impact of the laboratory environment on gamete and embryo quality. Reprod Biomed Online. 2014;28(3):198-203.
3. Magli MC, Van den Abbeel E, Lundin K, Royere D. Monitoring of air quality in the ART laboratory: A consensus guideline. Hum Reprod. 2016;31(7):1412-8.
4. Vermesh M, Samo M, Saadat P. Reducing contamination risks in ART: An evaluation of air quality and microbiological monitoring in IVF laboratories. Fertil Steril. 2020;113(3):519-29.

CHAPTER 3 Semen Analysis and Sperm Preparation

INTRODUCTION

Semen analysis and preparation form the bedrock of male fertility assessment and are essential steps in assisted reproductive technology (ART) procedures, such as intrauterine insemination (IUI), in-vitro fertilization (IVF), and intracytoplasmic sperm injection (ICSI). The primary goal of semen preparation is to isolate a highly motile, morphologically normal, and biochemically intact spermatozoa population free from seminal plasma and contaminants. Oxidative stress, a major contributor to sperm dysfunction, leads to increased DNA fragmentation, reduced motility, altered membrane integrity, and impaired fertilization potential. This stress may be intrinsic—originating from leukocytes or morphologically abnormal sperm—or extrinsic, caused by improper handling, repeated centrifugation, suboptimal pH, temperature fluctuations, or prolonged exposure to reactive oxygen species (ROS). Mitigation strategies include antioxidant-enriched media, strict temperature control, gentle centrifugation protocols, and minimal manipulation under sterile conditions.

In addition to cellular stress, psychological stress experienced by patients during semen collection can adversely affect ejaculatory function, volume, and semen quality. Factors such as anxiety, unfamiliar clinical environments, and time constraints can lead to suboptimal samples. To address this, clinics should provide private, comfortable, and stress-reducing collection areas, offer adequate preprocedural counseling, and, where necessary, allow home collection under controlled timelines with proper transport containers. Together, managing both biological and psychological stressors is essential to optimize sperm recovery and enhance ART outcomes.

SEMEN ANALYSIS

Semen is a composite fluid derived from multiple male reproductive glands, each contributing to its final composition. The sequential process of ejaculation begins with secretions from the Cowper's glands, which release a small volume of alkaline mucus-rich fluid for lubrication. This is followed by sperm-rich fluid from the epididymis and vas deferens (around 5–10% of total volume), which contains mature spermatozoa. The bulk of the ejaculate (60–70%) is contributed by the seminal vesicles, providing fructose, prostaglandins, and clotting factors. Finally, the prostate gland contributes about 20–30% of the volume, adding zinc, citric acid, and proteolytic enzymes essential for semen liquefaction. The precise timing and coordination of these secretions are crucial, as any alteration in the sequence such as incomplete or retrograde ejaculation—can affect sperm parameters and lead to misleading results.

For optimal reliability, semen collection should occur following 2–7 days of sexual abstinence. The sample should be collected by masturbation into a sterile, nontoxic, wide-mouthed container, preferably at the clinic to avoid temperature shifts and delays. If home collection is necessary, it must be delivered to the laboratory within 30–60 minutes, ensuring the sample is kept close to body temperature during transit. Analysis should ideally begin within 1 hour of collection, as delays may impact motility and viability due to increased oxidative stress and pH changes. Ensuring standardized collection and analysis protocols is essential for valid interpretation and for comparing results across cycles or clinics.

These parameters are critical in diagnosing male infertility and planning subsequent clinical procedures **(Table 1)**.

1. *Volume and liquefaction:* Normal ejaculate volume ranges from 1.5 to 5.0 mL, as defined by the World Health Organization. Deviations from this range can indicate disorders such as partial or total retrograde ejaculation, seminal vesicle dysfunction, or prolonged abstinence. Liquefaction, a process mediated by prostatic enzymes, should occur within 20–30 minutes after ejaculation. Delayed liquefaction, often due to prostatic infections or enzyme deficiencies, can be resolved using enzymatic treatments like α-chymotrypsin.[1]

TABLE 1: WHO Laboratory Manual for the Examination and Processing of Human Semen, 6th edition, 2021.

Parameter	*WHO 2021 reference value*
Volume	≥1.4 mL
Sperm concentration	≥16 million/mL
Total sperm count	≥39 million per ejaculate
Progressive motility (PR)	≥30%
Total motility (PR + NP)	≥42%
Morphology (normal forms and strict)	≥4%
Vitality (live sperm)	≥54%
pH	7.2–8.0
Leukocytes	<1 million/mL
Agglutination	None or occasional

2. *Sperm concentration and count:* Sperm concentration is determined using a hemocytometer or automated analyzers, with a normal value set at ≥15 million sperm/mL.[2] Low sperm concentration, known as oligozoospermia, can result from genetic anomalies, endocrine dysfunctions, or environmental factors.[3] Accurate concentration determination requires dilution and microscopic counting.
3. *Motility and vitality:* Sperm motility is categorized into progressive motility (PR), nonprogressive motility (NP), and immotility (IM). A sample is considered normal if it has ≥32% progressive motility. Factors influencing motility include oxidative stress, inappropriate handling during preparation, and infections.[4] Vitality, on the other hand, is assessed through hypoosmotic swelling (HOS) tests or eosin-nigrosin staining, where ≥58% live sperm is considered normal.[5]
4. *Morphology:* Sperm morphology evaluation using Kruger's strict criteria reveals that ≥4% normal forms are indicative of good fertilization potential.[6] Abnormal morphology can be due to testicular dysfunction, genetic defects (e.g., Y-chromosome microdeletions), or environmental insults.
5. *Presence of pus cells (leukocytes) and round cells:* Leukocytospermia, defined as >1 million leukocytes/mL, is associated with inflammation or infection, leading to increased ROS production that damages sperm DNA and impairs function.[7] Proper differentiation of leukocytes from immature germ cells can be achieved using peroxidase staining or monoclonal antibodies.
6. *Biochemical analysis:* Biochemical markers such as seminal fructose, citric acid, and zinc can provide insights into the functional status of the seminal vesicles, prostate, and epididymis. Deviations in these markers suggest glandular dysfunction and may aid in diagnosing accessory gland infections or obstructions.[8]

SEMEN PREPARATION TECHNIQUES

The purpose of semen preparation is to maximize the recovery of high-quality sperm while minimizing contamination and damage **(Table 2)**. The choice of technique depends on the initial quality of the semen sample, the specific ART procedure, and the presence of interfering substances like leukocytes or mucus **(Flowchart 1)**. In cases where density gradient centrifugation is employed, incomplete removal of

TABLE 2: Troubleshooting guide for semen analysis and preparation.

Issue	*Possible cause(s)*	*Solution*
High viscosity or delayed liquefaction	Inadequate liquefaction due to deficiency in prostatic enzymes, infection, or high mucous content	Use enzymatic treatment (e.g., α-chymotrypsin or bromelain) to facilitate liquefaction. Perform gentle pipetting to break down mucus. Optimize semen collection protocols to ensure complete liquefaction[2]
Low motility after preparation	Suboptimal centrifugation conditions, excessive mechanical stress, vibration or exposure to ROS during processing	Reduce centrifugation speed (200–300 g), shorten centrifugation time, and avoid prolonged exposure to ambient air. Use antioxidants (e.g., vitamin E and pentoxifylline) in washing media to reduce ROS damage[4]
Reduced sperm recovery post-preparation	Incomplete sample transfer, excessive force during resuspension, or over-centrifugation can result in significant sperm loss, particularly affecting fragile spermatozoa with compromised tail structures	Use calibrated wide-bore pipettes for viscous samples. Ensure gentle handling and use gravity force when resuspending pellets. Use lower centrifugal force and extended duration to improve recovery in difficult samples[2]
Pus cells or leukocytes trapping sperm	High leukocyte concentration leading to aggregation of pus cells and sperm	Use density gradient centrifugation to effectively separate sperm from leukocytes. Treat samples with anti-inflammatory agents or antibiotics as indicated. Incorporate MACS for additional isolation of high-quality sperm[7]
Agglutination of sperm (sperm clumping)	Presence of antisperm antibodies, high viscosity, or suboptimal preparation techniques	Treat samples with antibody removal media or use sperm wash buffer containing albumin. Perform density gradient centrifugation to reduce agglutination[4]
Excessive debris or nonsperm cells	Contamination from epithelial cells, leukocytes, or bacteria during collection or improper separation techniques	Optimize semen collection protocols and ensure sterile conditions. Use density gradient centrifugation to remove debris effectively[2]
Evaporation and pH changes in swim-up preparation	Dry incubator conditions, leading to pH and osmotic fluctuations in overlay media	Maintain humidity control within the incubator. Cover dishes with sterile oil or use closed systems to minimize evaporation. Pre-equilibrate media to stabilize pH before use[5]
Centrifuge-related pellet disturbance or low recovery	High-speed centrifugation or abrupt start/stop cycles causing shear stress and pellet loss	Use low-speed centrifugation (300–500 g), ensure smooth acceleration and deceleration settings, and balance tubes appropriately.[7] Perform a second wash with lower g-force to improve pellet stability

Contd...

Contd...

Issue	*Possible cause(s)*	*Solution*
Temperature-related sperm damage	Exposure to nonphysiological temperatures during sample handling or preparation, leading to loss of motility and vitality	Use temperature-controlled workstations and warm all handling equipment, including pipettes, tubes, and slides, to 37°C. Perform quick transfer between incubator and processing steps to minimize temperature fluctuations
Low recovery in microfluidic sperm selection	Suboptimal sample loading, improper device handling, or blockage of microchannels due to high viscosity	Dilute viscous samples before loading. Follow manufacturer's instructions for device setup and handling[10]
Low sperm recovery and quality during gradient preparation	Handling multiple OAT samples in separate tubes, improper pooling, clouding during resuspension, pellet disruption while layering, or physical stress to fragile sperm tails due to overcentrifugation or pipetting	For OAT cases, increase starting volume and use uniform discontinuous gradients across all tubes. Allow pellets to settle before pooling; avoid rapid mixing. While layering, pipette gently along the tube wall to prevent gradient disturbance. Centrifuge at recommended g-force (300–500 × g), avoid dry pellets, and gently resuspend to prevent tail breakage. Use wide-bore or soft-edged tips

(MACS: magnetic activated cell sorting; OAT: oligoasthenoteratozoospermia; ROS: reactive oxygen species)

Flowchart 1: Semen sample rejection and processing decision tree.

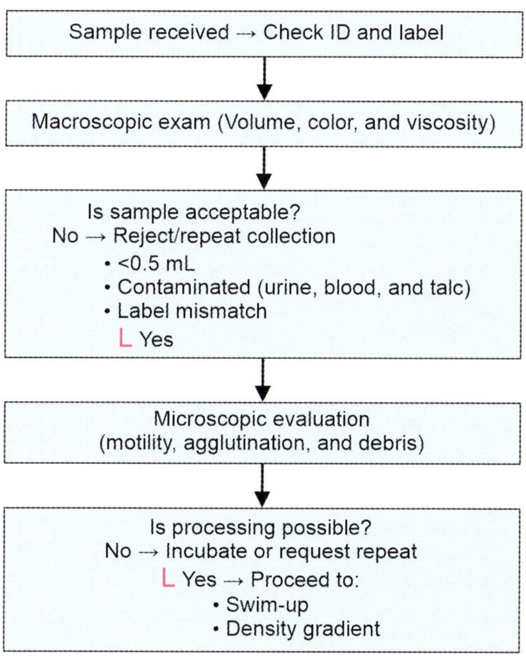

gradient media can compromise sperm function or lead to suboptimal embryo development. Therefore, careful aspiration of the sperm pellet and thorough washing are essential to avoid gradient carryover. Occasionally, visible granules or particulate debris may be observed in the final sample. It is advisable to allow the suspension to settle for a few minutes and then gently aspirate the top layer to ensure a cleaner fraction is used for insemination or injection.[2]

- *Simple wash method:* The simple wash method involves diluting semen with a washing medium, centrifuging to pellet sperm, and resuspending in fresh media. This technique is effective for normal or near-normal samples but can lead to sperm loss if not performed meticulously.[2] Over-centrifugation or excessive force during resuspension can damage sperm membranes, reducing motility and viability.[4]
- *Swim-up technique:* The swim-up method relies on motile sperm actively swimming into

an overlaid clean medium. While it is highly effective in isolating motile sperm, it is sensitive to pH and temperature changes, which can affect sperm function.[5] Modifications such as the use of gradient barriers or specialized chambers help to improve recovery.[2]

- *Density-gradient centrifugation:* Density-gradient centrifugation separates sperm based on density, enabling the isolation of highly motile, morphologically normal sperm.[7] This technique is ideal for samples with high debris or pus cells and is effective in eliminating dead sperm and other contaminants. Proper gradient layering and centrifuge settings are essential for optimal separation and yield.[4]
- *Advanced sperm selection methods:*
    - *Magnetic activated cell sorting (MACS):* This technique utilizes magnetic fields to separate apoptotic from nonapoptotic sperm, improving DNA integrity and reducing ROS levels.[9]
    - *Microfluidic sperm sorting:* A novel technique that provides a physiologically relevant environment for sperm selection based on motility, morphology, and DNA integrity. This method reduces oxidative damage and mechanical stress during preparation.[10]

CONCLUSION

Semen analysis and preparation are crucial steps in diagnosing and treating male infertility, as they provide essential insights into sperm quality and optimize samples for use in ART. Accurate analysis helps to identify potential issues such as low sperm count or poor motility, while proper preparation techniques, like density gradient centrifugation and swim-up, isolate the most viable sperm. Effective troubleshooting, such as managing viscosity or eliminating leukocytes, ensures high-quality sperm selection, which is essential for achieving optimal fertilization and improving ART outcomes. Adherence to established protocols and continuous refinement of techniques can significantly enhance clinical success rates and offer better chances of pregnancy for couples facing infertility.

REFERENCES

1. Zhang Z, Sun X, Wang L, Xu W, Wang Q. Seminal plasma proteins in semen analysis: An update. Clin Translat Med. 2020;10(2):70.
2. World Health Organization. WHO Laboratory Manual for the Examination and Processing of Human Semen, 6th edition. Geneva, Switzerland: WHO Press; 2021.
3. Sharma R, Harlev A, Agarwal A, Esteves SC. Cigarette smoking and semen quality: A new meta-analysis examining the effect of the 2010 World Health Organization laboratory methods for the examination of human semen. Eur Urol. 2018;74(5):626-37.
4. Agarwal A, Gupta S, Sharma R. Andrological Evaluation of Male Infertility: A Laboratory Guide. Berlin, Germany: Springer; 2016.
5. Esteves SC, Varghese AC, Agarwal A. Male Infertility: Contemporary Clinical Approaches, Andrology, ART and Antioxidants. Berlin, Germany: Springer; 2021.
6. Kruger TF, Acosta AA, Simmons KF, Swanson RJ, Matta JF, Oehninger S. Predictive value of abnormal sperm morphology in in vitro fertilization. Fertil Steril. 1988;49(1):112-7.
7. Henkel R, Kierspel E, Stalf T, Mehnert C, Menkveld R, Tinneberg HR, et al. Leukocytes and intrinsic ROS production do not influence sperm function. Andrologia. 2003;35(4):13-7.
8. Cooper TG, Noonan E, von Eckardstein S, Auger J, Baker HW, Behre HM, et al. World Health Organization reference values for human semen characteristics. Hum Reprod Update. 2010;16(3):231-45.
9. Pérez-Cerezales S, Boryshpolets S, Brand M. Proteomic changes in sperm during epididymal maturation. J Proteom. 2012;75(2):504-14.
10. Shirota K, Yotsumoto F, Itoh H, Obama H, Sato K. Separation efficiency of a microfluidic sperm sorter to minimize sperm DNA damage. Fertil Steril. 2016;105(2):315-21.

CHAPTER

4

Sperm Retrieval and Handling (Percutaneous Epididymal Sperm Aspiration, Testicular Sperm Aspiration, and Testicular Sperm Extraction)

INTRODUCTION

The management of azoospermia: whether obstructive azoospermia (OA) or nonobstructive azoospermia (NOA) has evolved significantly with the advent of microsurgical and percutaneous sperm retrieval techniques, which allow the acquisition of viable spermatozoa directly from the epididymis or testicular tissue. These procedures—namely "Percutaneous Epididymal Sperm Aspiration (PESA), Testicular Sperm Aspiration (TESA), and Testicular Sperm Extraction (TESE)" have become integral to assisted reproductive technology (ART), particularly when used in combination with intracytoplasmic sperm injection (ICSI) to overcome severe male factor infertility. However, these procedures are not without technical and biological challenges. The immature and fragile nature of surgically retrieved sperm, their limited motility, the risk of contamination with blood and cellular debris, and the complexities of cryopreservation make handling and processing in the laboratory a highly specialized task.

ANATOMICAL AND CLINICAL CONTEXT OF SPERM RETRIEVAL

Obstructive azoospermia results from congenital or acquired blockages in the reproductive tract, such as congenital bilateral absence of the vas deferens (CBAVD), vasectomy, or ejaculatory duct obstruction. In these cases, the testicular function is typically preserved, and motile sperm can often be retrieved from the epididymis using PESA. In contrast, NOA is a consequence of intrinsic testicular failure, often requiring TESE or micro-TESE for focal sperm retrieval.[1]

Percutaneous epididymal sperm aspiration is a relatively noninvasive procedure performed under local anesthesia, involving aspiration from the caput or corpus of the epididymis. TESA entails aspiration directly from the seminiferous tubules using a fine needle. TESE, including its microsurgical variant (micro-TESE), involves surgical dissection of testicular tissue to locate and extract areas of active spermatogenesis under an operating microscope **(Table 1)**.

LABORATORY HANDLING: ISOLATION, CONTAMINATION, AND PROCESSING

Immediately after retrieval, the sample is subjected to mechanical teasing or enzymatic digestion, especially for TESE, where sperm may be trapped within seminiferous tubules.[2] In cases of PESA or TESA, centrifugation is usually required to concentrate the sample, although this can inadvertently increase cell loss or pellet formation that traps nonmotile sperm. To prevent excessive dilution of the sperm count, it is advisable to use minimal culture media during sample collection and processing.

Microscopic identification of viable sperm in TESE or TESA samples often requires long search times and skilled personnel **(Table 2)**. Using phase contrast optics and enhanced contrast imaging can improve the efficiency of sperm retrieval.

TABLE 1: Comparative sperm yield, motility, morphology from PESA, TESA, and TESE.

Parameter	*PESA*	*TESA*	*TESE*
Source	Epididymal tubules	Testicular tissue (needle)	Testicular tissue (open biopsy)
Sperm yield	Moderate to high	Low to moderate	Variable, may be high (if tubules intact)
Motility	Good (progressive in many)	Poor to sluggish	Often nonmotile or sluggish
Morphology	Mature (elongated)	Immature (rounder and larger head)	Immature and heterogeneous
Debris/RBC load	Low to moderate	High	High
Cryosurvival	Good	Poor to moderate	Moderate
Complication risk	Minimal	Minimal	Higher (invasive procedure)

(PESA: percutaneous epididymal sperm aspiration; TESA: testicular sperm aspiration; TESE: testicular sperm extraction)

TABLE 2: Common laboratory issues and solutions in processing surgical samples.

Issue	*Mechanism*	*Impact*	*Solution*
Contamination with blood or fat	Rupture of surrounding capillaries or adipose	Interferes with sperm identification, increased ROS	Use density gradient centrifugation or erythrocyte lysis buffer[3]
Cell loss during processing	Adhesion to pipettes or incomplete recovery from dish	Reduced sperm availability for ICSI	Use low-adhesion pipette tips, rinse with sperm wash medium
Low motility or immotility	Intrinsic to testicular spermatozoa	Limits sperm selection and ICSI success	Use pentoxifylline or hypoosmotic swelling (HOS) test for viability
Presence of immature germ cells	Especially in NOA cases	Misidentification as sperm, debris overload	Training and experience in morphological identification are critical
Tissue fragments and viscosity	Post-TESE samples often contain sticky tissue remnants	Hinders isolation and smears micromanipulation field	Mechanical shredding using sterile needles or mincing with 26G needles

(ICSE: intracytoplasmic sperm injection; NOA: nonobstructive azoospermia; ROS: reactive oxygen species; TESE: testicular sperm extraction)

SPERM SELECTION AND VIABILITY ASSESSMENT

Unlike ejaculated sperm, testicular sperm are often nonmotile or show sluggish movement, making conventional selection techniques insufficient. Viability assessment becomes essential prior to ICSI.

Methods of Sperm Selection

- *Mechanical selection:* Based on subtle twitching, tail movement, or head-tail separation under 400×–600× magnification.
- *Hypoosmotic swelling (HOS) test:* Viable sperm will show tail curling in hypoosmotic solutions.[4]

- *Laser-assisted viability assessment:* An infrared laser pulse is directed at the sperm tail; viable sperm react with curling or movement.[5]
- *Chemical motility enhancers:* Agents like pentoxifylline (0.5–1 mM) may be used transiently to induce motility in dormant but viable sperm.[6] However, strict timing and washing are essential to avoid oocyte toxicity.

CRYOPRESERVATION AND THAWING OF SURGICALLY RETRIEVED SPERM

Cryopreserving testicular or epididymal sperm presents specific challenges due to the lower membrane integrity, limited numbers, and potential immaturity of retrieved cells.[7] Unlike ejaculated sperm, testicular sperms are more susceptible to cryodamage, leading to membrane disruption and loss of motility post-thaw.

Key Considerations in Cryopreservation

- *Cryoprotectants:* Glycerol-based media or commercial sperm freezing media with permeating and nonpermeating CPAs.
    - *Vial/Straw loading:* Sperm may be frozen in pellets, microdroplets, or straws with/without tissue, depending on sperm quantity.
    - *Cooling protocol:* Controlled slow freezing versus vitrification, recent evidence suggests vitrification may be superior in maintaining viability for immotile sperm.[7]
    - *Post-thaw recovery:* Samples must be handled gently; if motility is lost, HOS test or laser activation may again be required to assess viability before ICSI.

CLINICAL OUTCOMES AND PROGNOSTIC INDICATORS

Pregnancy outcomes using surgically retrieved sperm are largely dependent on the retrieval method, underlying testicular histopathology, and embryologist experience. While fertilization rates using PESA samples often approach those of ejaculated sperm, TESE samples: particularly from NOA patients tend to yield lower fertilization and blastocyst conversion rates due to intrinsic sperm defects.[1]

Predictive Markers of Successful Sperm Retrieval

- Presence of FSH <10 mIU/mL
- Normal testicular volume
- Histological diagnosis (e.g., hypospermatogenesis vs. Sertoli-cell-only syndrome)
- Detection of round spermatids or elongated spermatids indicating active spermatogenesis

TROUBLESHOOTING SPERM RETRIEVAL AND HANDLING

Surgically retrieved sperm present several unique challenges, including contamination with non-sperm cells, poor motility, immature morphology, and difficulties in cryopreservation.[2] These obstacles require embryologists to make real-time judgments to ensure viable sperm are efficiently isolated and used in ICSI **(Table 3)**.

SPECIFIC LABORATORY PRACTICES TO ENHANCE SPERM RECOVERY AND VIABILITY

- *Buffer optimization:*
    - Use HEPES-buffered media during microscopic examination to stabilize pH outside CO_2 incubators.
    - Incorporate antioxidants (e.g., taurine and hypotaurine) to mitigate oxidative stress in ROS-prone samples.
- *Centrifugation techniques:*
    - For PESA and TESA, use a mild centrifugation step (300 g for 10 minutes). Avoid high-speed spins which can damage fragile testicular sperm.

TABLE 3: Common troubleshooting issues in PESA/TESA/TESE handling.

Issue	*Scientific basis*	*Impact on ART*	*Recommended solution*
Contamination with RBCs and leukocytes	Disruption of blood vessels during biopsy leads to hemolysis and oxidative stress due to ROS release from WBCs	Impairs sperm viability, DNA integrity, and may introduce debris into ICSI field	Use erythrocyte lysis buffer or two-layer discontinuous density gradient to remove contaminants before sperm selection
Sperm adherence to dish or pipette	Protein-free culture media increase adherence, particularly in low-volume samples	Loss of rare spermatozoa during transfer; underestimation of sample potential	Use protein-supplemented medium (e.g., HSA or serum substitute supplement), rinse pipettes with medium containing 5% HSA
Fragmented tubules or tissue clumps post-TESE	Incomplete mechanical mincing releases few sperm trapped in seminiferous tubules	Low sperm yield despite good spermatogenesis	Use 26G needles for mincing, or enzymatic digestion with collagenase type IV followed by gentle centrifugation
Nonmotile sperm with intact morphology	Testicular sperm often lack motility due to immaturity or cryodamage but may still be viable	Difficult to assess suitability for ICSI	Perform HOS test or laser viability assay; use pentoxifylline temporarily for motility stimulation[6]
Identification errors due to cell debris	Co-presence of round cells (spermatids, and Sertoli cells) and germ-cell precursors	Leads to incorrect selection, risking failed fertilization	Training in morphology; use high magnification (400–600x) with Hoffman modulation contrast optics or IMSI
Poor post-thaw recovery	Intracellular ice formation damages plasma membrane; immature sperm more cryosensitive	Drastically reduced motility and membrane integrity	Prefer vitrification over slow freezing; avoid glycerol in immature sperm; use microdroplet freezing for single sperm[7]
Low yield despite clinical success	Sampling error in heterogeneous testicular tissue or inadequate biopsy depth	Misleadingly suggests failed retrieval	Consider repeat micro-TESE or deeper testicular biopsy under magnification
False negative results post-TESE	Failure to locate sperm due to poor sample preparation or inadequate search	Discarding potentially viable samples	Extend microscopic search time (>2 h), use overnight culture of tubule fragments to release late-recovering sperm
Cross-contamination during sample division or cryostorage	Shared cryotanks or open handling near other samples	Loss of patient's identity, medico-legal risk	Implement double witnessing, segregated cryostorage tanks, and labeled cryopreservation records with barcode verification

(ART: assisted reproductive technology; HSA: human serum albumin; ICSE: intracytoplasmic sperm injection; PESA: percutaneous epididymal sperm aspiration; ROS: reactive oxygen species; TESA: testicular sperm aspiration; TESE: testicular sperm extraction)

    - After centrifugation, examine both pellet and supernatant thoroughly for sperm presence before discarding.
- *Extended culture:* Short-term in vitro culture of testicular tissue at 34°C for 24 hours may enhance sperm motility and release from tubules in borderline samples.[3]
- *Use of microfluidics:* Emerging research supports using microfluidic sperm selection to separate sperm from debris and round cells with minimal physical handling, improving DNA integrity in surgically retrieved sperms.[4]

ADVANCED CRYOPRESERVATION STRATEGIES

Cryopreservation remains a challenge for surgically retrieved sperm due to low initial counts and their higher membrane fragility.

- *Microdroplet freezing:* For extremely low sperm numbers, loading 1–3 spermatozoa in 1 μL droplets on cryoloops or CryoTips improves post-thaw recovery.
- *Carrier-free vitrification:* Eliminates contamination risk and improves viability by vitrifying sperm in cell-safe carriers like closed-straw systems.[7]

CONCLUSION

Handling sperm retrieved via PESA, TESA, or TESE requires a detailed understanding of male reproductive anatomy, pathophysiology of azoospermia, and specialized laboratory techniques tailored to low-volume and low-motility samples. From avoiding contamination to identifying viable immotile sperm, and from cryopreservation to optimizing ICSI outcomes, embryologists must employ precise methods and maintain stringent quality controls. With increasing use of PGT and fertility preservation, optimizing surgical sperm retrieval protocols remains a vital pillar in reproductive medicine.

REFERENCES

1. Schlegel PN. Testicular sperm extraction: microdissection improves sperm yield with minimal tissue excision. Hum Reprod. 1999;14(1):131-5.
2. Schlegel PN, Su LM, Goldstein M. Microsurgical TESE: Technical aspects and results. Urolog Clin North Am. 1999;25(4):677-88.
3. Esteves SC, Miyaoka R, Agarwal A. An update on the clinical assessment of the infertile male. Clinics. 2011;66(4):691-700.
4. World Health Organization. WHO laboratory manual for the examination and processing of human semen, 6th edition. Geneva: WHO Press; 2021.
5. Aktan TM, Montag M, Diedrich K. Laser-assisted immotile sperm selection for ICSI. Hum Reprod. 2004;19(3):623-7.
6. Dozortsev D, Rybouchkin A, De Sutter P, Dhont M. Sperm viability test using the hypo-osmotic swelling test. Hum Reprod. 1995;10(1):196-200.
7. Isachenko V, Isachenko E, Montag M, Zaeva V, Krivokharchenko A, Katkov II, et al. Vitrification of human spermatozoa: a step towards a new era of sperm cryopreservation. Reproductive Biomedicine Online. 2008;17(4):510-5.

CHAPTER 5

Oocyte Cumulus Complex Scanning

INTRODUCTION

Oocyte cumulus complex (OCC) scanning is a critical step in assessing oocyte quality and predicting developmental potential in assisted reproductive technology (ART) laboratories. Embryologists carefully examine the cumulus cell expansion, oocyte visibility, and cytoplasmic clarity, while also noting the composition and appearance of follicular fluid. Ideal follicular fluid is clear to slightly yellow, while the presence of blood clots, excessive granulosa cell debris, or dense turbidity may indicate trauma or suboptimal aspiration technique, which can compromise oocyte health.[1] The presence of dark brown fluid or foul odor may reflect endometriosis or infection. Additionally, the degree of cumulus expansion, from compact to fully expanded, reflects the oocyte's maturity and responsiveness to luteinizing hormone (LH) surge or human chorionic gonadotropin (hCG) trigger.[2] Abnormally thin cumulus or absent corona radiata may suggest atresia or incomplete maturation.[3] Blood-stained or highly viscous samples can obscure oocyte detection and increase the risk of missing viable oocytes. Therefore, accurate scanning with gentle rotation of the collection tube and minimizing blood contamination are essential to preserve the integrity and viability of oocytes for downstream procedures like intracytoplasmic sperm injection (ICSI) or in-vitro fertilization (IVF).[4]

UNDERSTANDING OOCYTE CUMULUS COMPLEX MORPHOLOGY

The OCC comprises the oocyte surrounded by multiple layers of cumulus granulosa cells. The morphology of these cumulus cells and the oocyte itself is indicative of oocyte health and developmental potential. Key characteristics to observe during OCC scanning include:

Cumulus Expansion and Cell Layers

A healthy oocyte is generally surrounded by several layers of expanded cumulus cells. The degree of cumulus expansion is directly influenced by oocyte maturation and can vary depending on hormonal stimulation and oocyte developmental stage.[5]

Oocyte Size and Shape

Normal oocytes typically measure 110–120 µm in diameter, with a uniform cytoplasm and clear zona pellucida. Deviations from this size or the presence of abnormalities such as cytoplasmic granularity or vacuoles can indicate compromised oocyte quality.[6]

Cumulus Matrix and Mucification

The cumulus matrix, enriched in hyaluronic acid and proteoglycans, should appear clear and gelatinous. A thick, sticky, or highly dense matrix can impair oocyte release during denudation, complicating subsequent ICSI procedures.[7]

Accurate identification of abnormalities during OCC and follicular fluid scanning requires not only observational expertise but also a deep understanding of the physiological, mechanical, and chemical factors that influence OCC morphology. Factors such as stimulation protocols, follicular environment, enzymatic exposure, and handling conditions can significantly affect the cumulus expansion, matrix texture, and oocyte visibility. Additionally, the composition of follicular fluid ranging from its color and clarity to the presence of blood, pus, or granulosa tissue serves as a window into the follicle's health and directly correlates with oocyte quality and developmental potential.[8] Recognizing these variations and implementing corrective strategies is crucial for optimizing fertilization, minimizing oocyte loss, and ensuring consistent laboratory outcomes. The following table summarizes common issues encountered during OCC and follicular fluid scanning, their possible causes, impact on ART outcomes, and evidence-based solutions **(Table 1)**.

TABLE 1: Troubleshooting guide for oocyte cumulus complex (OCC) and follicular fluid scanning.

Issue	*Possible cause(s)*	*Impact on ART outcomes*	*Solution*
Thin cumulus layer or minimal expansion	Low FSH or LH stimulation, premature oocyte retrieval, or inadequate preovulatory hormonal support[7]	Reduced maturation potential, lower fertilization rates, and poor embryo quality	Increasing gonadotropin doses in subsequent cycles. Adjust timing of retrieval to ensure oocyte maturity. Consider the use of rescue in-vitro maturation (IVM) for immature oocytes to enhance their developmental competence
Large, expanded cumulus but with no oocyte (empty follicle)	Improper follicular aspiration technique, suboptimal timing, or luteinized unruptured follicles can lead to the retrieval of empty follicles or missed oocytes during aspiration; in some cases, even an empty zona pellucida may be observed, indicating oocyte extrusion or degeneration prior to retrieval[9]	Missed oocyte retrieval and potential reduction in the number of fertilizable oocytes	Carefully scan follicular fluid in search for missed oocytes. Adjust aspiration technique to ensure all potential sites are aspirated. Consider a second-look aspiration if no oocyte is recovered from a follicle. Evaluate timing of oocyte retrieval relative to hCG or GnRH agonist trigger. Implement ultrasound guidance if needed
Presence of granulosa cells and pus cells in follicular fluid	Infection or inflammation within the follicle, improper collection techniques, or contamination during sample processing can compromise oocyte quality and retrieval outcomes; in some instances, the presence of ovarian stromal tissue or granulosa-luteinized cell clumps in the aspirate may further indicate disrupted follicular architecture or an overly aggressive aspiration approach[5]	Increased ROS production, impaired oocyte quality, and lower fertilization potential	Assess follicular fluid for signs of infection or inflammation. Use leukocyte peroxidase staining or microbiological testing to confirm presence of infection. Implement additional follicular washing steps to remove inflammatory cells. Consider antibiotic treatment if infection is confirmed

Contd...

Contd...

Issue	*Possible cause(s)*	*Impact on ART outcomes*	*Solution*
Blood contamination in follicular fluid	Excessive aspiration pressure, use of sharp needles, or follicle wall damage during retrieval[10]	Increased oxidative stress, impaired visualization, and compromised oocyte quality	Adjust aspiration pressure and use rounded-tip needles to reduce trauma. Avoid over-aspiration of follicles and monitor the fluid for signs of hemorrhage. Perform an extra wash to remove blood cells before further handling. Utilize anticoagulants or media additives to reduce oxidative stress induced by hemoglobin release
Air bubbles in follicular fluid or OCC	Improper pipetting technique, introduction of air during collection or transfer, or suboptimal handling conditions[11]	Mechanical disruption of cumulus cells, interference with ICSI procedures, and impaired visualization	Pre-equilibrate media and ensure pipettes are free of air before transfer. Use controlled pipetting techniques and avoid rapid pipetting. Remove air bubbles by allowing them to settle or by using a micropipette to gently aspirate them without disturbing the OCC. Ensure tubes and pipettes are properly sealed to prevent air entry during fluid handling
Thick and sticky OCCs difficult to denude	Excessive hyaluronic acid production due to hyperstimulation, abnormal follicular fluid composition, or suboptimal enzymatic treatment during denudation[8]	Difficulties in oocyte isolation, increased risk of mechanical damage, and lower ICSI efficiency	Use enzymatic treatments (e.g., hyaluronidase) at appropriate concentrations for a controlled duration to break down the cumulus matrix. Adjust stimulation protocols to reduce hyperstimulation and prevent excessive hyaluronic acid production. Utilize gentle pipetting during denudation to avoid oocyte damage. Perform a second round of light enzyme treatment if necessary
Collapsed or flattened cumulus matrix	Excessive mechanical force during aspiration or handling, improper denudation technique, or chemical contamination in the medium	Increased mechanical stress, lower oocyte viability, and reduced fertilization potential	Use soft pipetting techniques and minimal suction force during aspiration and denudation. Limit exposure to denuding media and avoid harsh pipetting. Ensure all media and consumables are free from contaminants. Use wide-bore pipettes to minimize shear forces and avoid collapsing the cumulus matrix

Contd...

Contd...

Issue	*Possible cause(s)*	*Impact on ART outcomes*	*Solution*
OCCs with mucus or gelatinous substance	High viscosity of follicular fluid due to hormonal imbalance or contamination from cervical mucus during collection	Increased difficulty in oocyte isolation, reduced efficiency of enzymatic treatments, and potential contamination of culture media	Perform additional washes to dilute and remove mucus. Use gentle pipetting to disperse mucus without causing damage to the cumulus matrix. Avoid contamination from the cervical area during sample collection by ensuring the catheter is properly positioned in the follicle. Consider enzymatic treatment to reduce viscosity if mucus persists
Delayed cumulus expansion postretrieval	Inadequate preovulatory hormone levels, inappropriate timing of oocyte retrieval, or compromised cumulus cell function[7]	Reduced cumulus-oocyte signaling, lower maturation potential, and impaired fertilization outcomes	Assess hormonal levels (FSH and LH) and consider adjusting dosages in future cycles. Extend in-vitro maturation (IVM) time if needed to allow for complete cumulus expansion. Supplement culture medium with growth factors like EGF (epidermal growth factor) to promote cumulus expansion and support oocyte maturation
Presence of small, fragmented cumulus clumps	Overexposure to enzymatic treatments, mechanical stress during handling, or inadequate culture conditions	Fragmented cumulus indicates reduced viability of the complex and lower developmental potential	Minimize exposure to hyaluronidase and use gentle handling techniques to prevent mechanical fragmentation. Use minimal mechanical force during aspiration and denudation to preserve cumulus integrity. Consider using mechanical denudation methods rather than prolonged enzymatic treatment. Adjust culture conditions to ensure optimal cumulus cell health
Oocyte or cumulus complex dislodged from dish during handling	Improper aspiration or pipetting techniques, inadequate dish design, or overfilled medium leading to turbulence during handling	Loss of oocytes, increased handling time, and reduced accuracy during ICSI or micromanipulation	Use dishes with appropriate well sizes and ensure optimal medium volume. Avoid overfilling culture dishes. Use controlled pipetting techniques to minimize turbulence. Implement steady and gentle movements during handling to avoid accidental dislodgment of oocytes. If an oocyte is dislodged, recover it promptly using a soft-tip pipette and minimize additional handling to preserve quality

Contd...

Contd...

Issue	*Possible cause(s)*	*Impact on ART outcomes*	*Solution*
Dark or discolored oocyte cytoplasm	Suboptimal follicular environment, high oxidative stress, or genetic abnormalities affecting cytoplasmic quality[2]	Poor oocyte quality, lower fertilization potential, and compromised embryo development	Evaluate follicular fluid and environment for oxidative stress markers or metabolic imbalances. Use antioxidants in culture media to support cytoplasmic health. Consider excluding oocytes with severe discoloration from ICSI. If persistent, investigate possible genetic causes and consider advanced diagnostic techniques to determine underlying pathology
OCCs with unusually hard or rigid matrix	Chemical contamination, oxidative stress, or suboptimal follicular microenvironment during oocyte maturation[8]	Difficulty in processing, impaired handling during ICSI, and potential oocyte damage	Use antioxidants and pH stabilizers in the culture medium if oxidative stress is suspected. Ensure all media and consumables are free from chemical contaminants. Optimize stimulation protocols to promote a balanced follicular environment. Consider using milder enzymatic treatment or mechanical denudation techniques to handle rigid cumulus complexes with minimal damage. Regularly check and calibrate equipment to ensure the maintenance of ideal culture conditions

(ART: assisted reproductive technology; FSH: follicle-stimulating hormone; GnRH: gonadotropin-releasing hormone; hCG: human chorionic gonadotropin; ICSI: intracytoplasmic sperm injection; LH: luteinizing hormone; ROS: reactive oxygen species)

CONCLUSION

Oocyte cumulus complex and follicular fluid scanning are vital aspects of oocyte quality assessment in IVF laboratories. The ability to recognize and resolve issues such as poor cumulus expansion, blood contamination, and abnormal matrix consistency is essential for optimizing fertilization outcomes and ensuring high-quality oocyte selection. By implementing targeted troubleshooting strategies based on an embryologist's perspective, it is possible to improve handling efficiency, enhance ICSI success rates, and contribute to better clinical outcomes for patients undergoing fertility treatment.

REFERENCES

1. Fatemi HM, Kyrou D, Bourgain C, Van den Abbeel E, Griesinger G, Devroey P. Cryopreserved-thawed human embryos transferred at the blastocyst stage: Relationship to embryo quality and woman's age. Hum Reprod. 2006;21(3):595-9.

2. Mikkelsen AL, Lindenberg S. Benefit of FSH priming of women with PCOS to oocyte maturation and embryo quality. Hum Reprod. 2001;16(6):1152-6.
3. Eppig JJ. Oocyte control of ovarian follicular development and function in mammals. Reproduction. 2020;159(3):F1-17.
4. Combelles CM, Cekleniak NA, Racowsky C, Albertini DF. Assessment of nuclear and cytoplasmic maturation in in-vitro matured human oocytes. Hum Reprod. 2002;17(4):1006-16.
5. Hyttel P, Sinowatz F, Vejlsted M. Essentials of domestic animal embryology. Amsterdam, Netherlands: Elsevier Health Sciences; 2018.
6. Van Blerkom J. Mitochondria in human oogenesis and preimplantation embryogenesis: Engines of metabolism, ionic regulation and developmental competence. Reproduction. 2008;128(3): 269-80.
7. Li R, Jin L, Ma X, Zhang Y, Zhang J. Maternal control of oocyte quality in mammals. Reprod Biol Endocrinol. 2017;15(1):68.
8. Swain JE, Carrell D, Racowsky C. Optimizing embryo culture conditions. Cambridge: Cambridge University Press; 2016.
9. Swain JE. Optimizing the culture environment in the IVF laboratory: Impact of pH and buffer capacity on gamete and embryo quality. Reprod Biomed Online. 2010;21(1):6-16.
10. Balaban B, Urman B, Sertac A, Alatas C, Aksoy S, Mercan R. Oocyte morphology does not predict fertilization rate, embryo quality, and implantation rate after intracytoplasmic sperm injection. Fertil Steril. 2011;76(5):928-31.
11. Ndukwe G, Thornton S, Fishel S, Alfirevic Z, Taylor A. Empty follicle syndrome: Successful treatment in subsequent cycles. Hum Reprod. 1996;11(1):39-41.

CHAPTER

6 Oocyte Denudation

INTRODUCTION

Oocyte denudation is a critical laboratory process that involves the meticulous removal of cumulus and corona radiata cells surrounding the oocyte. This procedure is essential for preparing the oocyte for intracytoplasmic sperm injection (ICSI) and for conducting a thorough assessment of oocyte morphology, as the removal of these cells reveals the zona pellucida, allowing for direct visualization and evaluation of the oocyte's maturity and structural integrity. The denudation process relies on a delicate balance of enzymatic digestion using hyaluronidase and mechanical manipulation with specialized pipettes. Hyaluronidase facilitates the breakdown of the extracellular matrix composed of hyaluronic acid, making it easier to dislodge the cumulus cells, while gentle pipetting ensures that the surrounding cumulus and corona cells are effectively removed without causing mechanical trauma to the oocyte. The objective is to achieve complete removal of the cumulus cells while maintaining the oocyte's structural integrity and ensuring that the zona pellucida remains intact and undamaged.

If the denudation procedure is not executed with precision whether due to overexposure to enzymatic treatment, inappropriate pipetting force, or incorrect handling techniques can result in detrimental effects such as thinning or tearing of the zona pellucida, cytoplasmic extrusion, or even complete loss of the oocyte. These adverse outcomes can subsequently compromise oocyte quality, reduce fertilization rates, and negatively impact embryonic development. Therefore, it is imperative that embryologists maintain strict control over each aspect of the denudation process, including enzyme concentration, exposure time, pipette diameter, and mechanical force, to safeguard oocyte viability and optimize assisted reproductive technology (ART) outcomes.

TECHNICAL ASPECTS OF OOCYTE CUMULUS COMPLEX DENUDATION

- *Enzymatic treatment:*
    - *Hyaluronidase concentration and exposure time:* The hyaluronic acid matrix surrounding the oocyte is digested using hyaluronidase enzyme, which facilitates the removal of cumulus cells. A concentration of 40–80 IU/mL is commonly used, with an exposure time of 30 seconds to 2 minutes depending on the density and consistency of the cumulus matrix.[1] Excessive exposure time or high enzyme concentration can cause damage to the zona pellucida and increase the risk of oocyte degeneration.[2] It is essential to monitor the oocytes under a microscope during the process to assess cumulus removal efficiency and oocyte morphology.
- *Capillary diameter:*
    - The diameter of the denuding pipette plays a pivotal role in the safety and effectiveness of the denudation process. Pipette diameters typically range from 120 to 180 μm for initial removal of cumulus cells and

100–120 μm for final denudation of the corona radiata cells.[3] Using a capillary with an inappropriate diameter can result in mechanical stress, incomplete removal of cumulus cells, or oocyte damage. For fragile oocytes, it is recommended to use a slightly larger diameter initially to minimize mechanical stress, followed by a smaller diameter for fine removal of residual cells.

- *Mechanical pipetting force:* Mechanical denudation is performed using repetitive, gentle pipetting to shear off remaining cumulus and corona cells. Excessive force or rapid pipetting can result in cytoplasmic extrusion, zona pellucida fractures, or disintegration of fragile oocytes.[4] The pipetting force should be adjusted based on the viscosity of the medium and the size and fragility of the oocyte.
- *Media selection and handling conditions:* The denudation medium should be equilibrated to physiological temperature (37°C) and pH (7.2–7.4) to maintain oocyte health. The medium should also have low viscosity to facilitate smooth removal of cumulus cells without inducing shear stress. The use of media with antioxidants, such as L-glutathione, can reduce oxidative stress during denudation and improve oocyte outcomes.[5]
- *Handling and timing:* Minimize oocyte exposure to ambient conditions to prevent temperature and pH fluctuations. The entire denudation process, including enzymatic treatment and mechanical pipetting, should not exceed 5–7 minutes to prevent prolonged exposure and potential damage to oocyte quality.[5] Group denudation, though time-efficient in high-volume laboratories, may pose a higher risk of oocyte mix-up or uneven enzymatic exposure. On the other hand, individual denudation allows for more controlled handling and traceability. Ultimately, both methods can yield excellent outcomes when performed by skilled embryologists with precise coordination, adherence to SOPs, and awareness of time-sensitivity and aseptic technique **(Table 1)**.

TABLE 1: Schematic comparison of enzymatic versus mechanical denudation.

Parameter	*Enzymatic denudation*	*Mechanical denudation*
Objective	Loosen cumulus-corona cells using enzyme	Remove residual cells using pipetting
Key material	Hyaluronidase enzyme (80 IU/mL)	IVF grade media, fine denudation pipette
Pipette size	Wide bore (200 μm)	Narrow bore (≤140 μm)
Timeframe	≤30 seconds exposure to enzyme	2–5 minutes depending on batch size
Step 1	Pipette OCCs gently 2–3x in hyaluronidase drop	Pipette denuded oocytes 4–6x in washing drop
Step 2	Transfer immediately to washing drop to stop enzyme	Examine oocytes under inverted microscope
Step 3	Begin mechanical denudation	Final rinse before ICSI
Precaution	Avoid prolonged exposure (>60 seconds) to prevent zona damage	Avoid excessive pipetting to maintain cytoplasmic integrity
Endpoint check	Cumulus cells loosened, but corona may remain	Clear zona, polar body visible, ooplasm intact

(ICSI: intracytoplasmic sperm injection; OCC: oocyte cumulus complex)

- *Cleaning and equipment maintenance:* All capillaries, pipettes, and handling dishes should be thoroughly cleaned and sterilized before use. Residual chemicals or contaminants can lead to impaired denudation and damage to the oocyte. Regular calibration of pipetting forces and inspection of pipettes for any structural defects are critical to ensure the integrity and safety of the denudation process.

TROUBLESHOOTING DURING OOCYTE CUMULUS COMPLEX DENUDATION

The denudation process involves several delicate steps that require careful attention to detail. Improper technique or suboptimal conditions can lead to various issues, impacting the quality and developmental potential of the oocyte. **Table 2** provides a comprehensive troubleshooting guide that addresses common problems encountered

TABLE 2: Troubleshooting guide for oocyte cumulus complex (OCC) denudation.

Issue	*Possible cause(s)*	*Impact on ART outcomes*	*Solution*
Excessive time in hyaluronidase solution	Incorrect concentration of enzyme, prolonged exposure due to difficult removal of cumulus cells, or inadequate mixing of enzyme solution	Damage to zona pellucida integrity, impaired oocyte quality, and increased risk of cytoplasmic damage	Use a concentration of 80 IU/mL hyaluronidase and limit exposure time to 30–60 seconds. Monitor denudation under a microscope to ensure timely removal of the cumulus. Transfer the oocytes to fresh handling medium immediately after denudation. Confirm enzyme effectiveness through batch testing
Fragile or collapsing oocytes	Mechanical stress during pipetting, high suction force, or prolonged exposure to enzyme leading to zona pellucida weakening	Zona fracture, cytoplasmic leakage, or oocyte fragmentation, leading to poor ICSI outcomes	Use gentle pipetting techniques with wide-bore pipettes to minimize mechanical stress. Avoid prolonged enzyme exposure to prevent weakening of the zona. Reduce suction force during pipetting and monitor for signs of cytoplasmic leakage. Modify enzyme concentration by serial dilution or exposure time based on OCC condition
Presence of air bubbles in the capillary or media	Improper pipetting technique, air introduced during loading or transfer, or inadequate equilibration of media	Disruption of oocyte structure, increased risk of mechanical damage, and interference with visual assessment	Ensure that all pipettes and capillaries are pre-equilibrated and bubble-free before use. Use slow and steady pipetting to minimize air entry. Remove any visible bubbles using a micropipette without disturbing the oocyte. Consider using capillaries with bubble-trapping designs to avoid introducing air during handling

Contd...

Contd...

Issue	*Possible cause(s)*	*Impact on ART outcomes*	*Solution*
Loss of oocytes during denudation	Excessive pipetting force, use of a capillary with an inappropriate diameter, or overexposure to enzyme causing zona pellucida thinning	Reduced yield of oocytes for ICSI, increased risk of losing high-quality oocytes, and poor treatment outcomes	Use appropriate capillary diameters (120–180 µm for initial denudation and 100–120 µm for final denudation). Employ soft-pipetting techniques and monitor oocytes carefully during denudation. If oocyte loss is frequent, reassess enzyme exposure times and mechanical force applied during denudation
Leftover media in the capillary	Improper flushing of the capillary before use or inadequate control during pipetting, leading to inconsistent media volume in the capillary	Introduction of air into the system, inconsistent removal of cumulus cells, and impaired visualization	Thoroughly flush the capillary with handling medium before use. Use consistent pipetting techniques to ensure proper filling of the capillary with no leftover media. Regularly check capillaries for blockage or media retention and replace as necessary. Consider using microcapillaries with optimized flow control for consistent denudation
Turbidity in the denudation medium	Contamination from cumulus cell debris, excessive enzyme presence, or inadequate washing postdenudation	Impaired visualization during denudation, difficulty in identifying and isolating oocytes, and risk of contamination	Use an additional washing step after denudation to remove cumulus cell debris and enzyme residues. Replace the denudation medium frequently to maintain clarity and ensure optimal conditions. Use fresh medium for each batch of denuded oocytes to avoid contamination and debris accumulation. Avoid overloading dishes with multiple OCCs during denudation
Oocytes adhering to the capillary walls	High viscosity of medium, suboptimal pipetting force, or inappropriate capillary diameter	Increased risk of mechanical damage, inconsistent cumulus removal, and loss of oocytes during transfer	Use low-viscosity media for denudation and ensure optimal medium volume in the capillary. Use gentle pipetting and a consistent flow rate during denudation. Opt for capillary diameters appropriate for the size and type of oocyte complex being handled. Consider precoating capillaries with handling medium to reduce oocyte adherence

Contd...

Contd...

Issue	*Possible cause(s)*	*Impact on ART outcomes*	*Solution*
Oocyte rotation or displacement during pipetting	Inconsistent pipetting force, use of inappropriate pipette tip, or mechanical stress from surrounding cells or debris	Displacement of oocytes, increased handling time, and risk of oocyte loss	Ensure gentle and consistent pipetting with minimal mechanical stress. Use a pipette tip suitable for the size of the oocyte to maintain control during denudation. Consider using a holding pipette to stabilize the oocyte during final denudation steps. Utilize a temperature-controlled microscope stage to maintain stable environmental conditions during denudation
Persistent cumulus cell clumps adhering to the oocyte	Incomplete enzymatic digestion of cumulus cells, low enzyme concentration, or inadequate mechanical pipetting	Residual cumulus cells may hinder ICSI, increase mechanical stress during injection, and reduce fertilization rates.	Increase enzyme concentration slightly or extend exposure time under careful observation. Use gentle mechanical pipetting to remove remaining cumulus cells without damaging the oocyte. Consider using an additional round of mild enzyme treatment if clumps persist. Regularly calibrate pipetting forces and ensure uniform application during denudation
Oocyte turbidity or cloudiness postdenudation	Chemical contamination in the media, exposure to nonphysiological temperatures, or oxidative damage during handling	Reduced oocyte quality, lower fertilization rates, and compromised embryo development	Assess media and consumables for potential contaminants. Use antioxidants in the handling medium if oxidative stress is suspected. Ensure that all handling and denudation procedures are performed at 37°C and within pH-controlled conditions. Utilize a closed environment to minimize exposure to ambient air and potential contaminants
Delayed or incomplete denudation	Low enzyme concentration, inadequate exposure time, or improper mechanical pipetting technique	Presence of residual cumulus cells, increased risk of damage during ICSI, and lower fertilization rates	Optimize hyaluronidase concentration and exposure time. Use a consistent mechanical pipetting technique with gradual force. If residual cells persist, repeat enzyme treatment with adjusted parameters. Consider mechanical denudation using a holding pipette and appropriate capillary diameters for complete removal of cumulus cells

Contd...

Contd...

Issue	*Possible cause(s)*	*Impact on ART outcomes*	*Solution*
Hard or rigid cumulus matrix	Chemical contamination, oxidative stress, or inadequate follicular support during oocyte maturation	Difficulty in removing cumulus cells, risk of mechanical damage during denudation, and poor oocyte quality	Use antioxidants and pH stabilizers in the culture medium if oxidative stress is suspected. Ensure media and consumables are free from contaminants. Modify stimulation protocols to optimize the follicular environment and support proper cumulus matrix development. Consider mechanical denudation with minimal enzymatic treatment to reduce mechanical stress on rigid cumulus complexes
Accidental contact with sperm drops during oocyte loading	Inattentive pipetting technique, dish overcrowding, improper layout of droplets, or shaky hand movement during oocyte transfer to the ICSI dish	Risk of unintentional sperm exposure to oocytes before ICSI, possible polyspermy, zona hardening due to premature sperm contact, or unidentified fertilization prior to controlled insemination. May also increase mechanical stress on oocytes	Redesign the dish layout to maintain adequate distance between PVP drop and oocyte drops. Train personnel on ergonomic pipetting angles and steady hand technique. Always label and predefine sperm and oocyte drop positions. Use a fresh dish if cross-contamination is suspected. Reinforce slow, controlled movements during oocyte loading to avoid pipette drift or accidental contact

(ICSI: intracytoplasmic sperm injection; PVP: polyvinylpyrrolidone)

during OCC denudation, their underlying causes, and suggested solutions to improve the outcomes of the denudation process.

CONCLUSION

Oocyte cumulus complex denudation is a technically sensitive and biologically critical procedure that directly influences the success of ICSI and subsequent embryonic development. Ensuring optimal outcomes requires a precise combination of enzymatic and mechanical methods tailored to the characteristics of each oocyte cohort. From enzyme concentration and exposure timing to pipette diameter and media selection, every variable plays a vital role in safeguarding oocyte viability. Furthermore, meticulous technique, vigilant observation, and timely troubleshooting are essential in minimizing cellular damage, contamination, or handling errors. Regular training, calibration, and adherence to validated protocols help to maintain consistency, reduce variability, and enhance the overall efficiency and safety of the ART laboratory. Ultimately, a well-executed denudation process contributes significantly to fertilization success and the potential for viable embryo formation.

REFERENCES

1. Hyttel P, Fair T, Callesen H, Greve T. Oocyte growth, capacitation, and final maturation in cattle. Theriogenology. 2018;49(1):23-32.
2. Wang X, Yin H. The impact of hyaluronidase concentration on human oocyte morphology and fertilization rates. Fertil Steril. 2019;98(3):598-603.
3. Esteves SC, Varghese AC, Agarwal A. Practical Manual of In Vitro Fertilization: Advanced Methods and Novel Devices. New York: Springer; 2021.
4. Esfandiari N, Arici A. In vitro assessment of oocyte quality and maturation. Reprod BioMed Online. 2020;15(5):545-53.
5. Parmegiani L, Cognigni GE, Bernardi S, Troilo E, Maccarini G. Comparison of two hyaluronidase preparations in denuding cumulus-oocyte complexes for intracytoplasmic sperm injection: evaluation of denudation time, oocyte morphology, and embryo quality. J Assist Reprod Genetics. 2014;31(4):463-9.

CHAPTER 7

Oocyte Assessment

INTRODUCTION

Oocyte quality plays a crucial role in determining the success of fertilization, embryo development, and eventual pregnancy outcomes in assisted reproductive technology (ART). As the largest cell in the human body, the oocyte contributes not only half of the genetic material but also the entirety of the mitochondria that power the early embryo until embryonic genome activation occurs. This maternal contribution extends beyond nuclear DNA to include epigenetic regulators, organelles, transcripts, and cytoplasmic reserves essential for early cleavage and embryonic competence. Evaluating oocyte quality requires a detailed analysis of multiple morphological and biochemical parameters, including cumulus cell integrity, polar body (PB) morphology, cytoplasmic characteristics, and zona pellucida (ZP) structure.[1] Each of these factors offers valuable insights into the oocyte's capacity to achieve successful fertilization and support early embryonic development. Any anomalies present in these characteristics—such as cytoplasmic vacuoles, lipid accumulation, perivitelline (PV) space debris, or smooth endoplasmic reticulum clusters (SERCs)—can lead to developmental arrest, poor implantation potential, and increased risk of aneuploidy or chromosomal abnormalities. Understanding the significance of these parameters and identifying common issues enable embryologists to troubleshoot effectively. Addressing these concerns and implementing corrective strategies ensures the selection of high-quality oocytes for ART procedures, ultimately enhancing clinical outcomes and improving the likelihood of successful pregnancy.

MORPHOLOGICAL ASSESSMENT OF CUMULUS-OOCYTE COMPLEX

The cumulus-oocyte complex (COC) is an essential structure that supports the maturation and protection of the oocyte. Cumulus cells form multiple layers surrounding the oocyte, providing it with critical nutrients, growth factors, and signaling molecules that facilitate nuclear and cytoplasmic maturation. The degree of cumulus cell expansion and the overall morphology of the COC serve as valuable indicators of oocyte developmental competence **(Table 1)**.[2-4] Optimal follicular aspiration is vital to preserve the integrity of the COC and to retrieve high-quality oocytes. To maintain the native environment of the oocyte, follicular fluid should be collected without the use of flushing, which may reduce the concentration of essential proteins and growth factors. The use of saline or phosphate-buffered solutions for flushing is discouraged, as these lack the biochemical components found in natural follicular fluid. Furthermore, efforts should be made to minimize blood contamination during aspiration, as hemoglobin and inflammatory mediators present in blood can be toxic to oocytes. Instead, obtaining undiluted, clear follicular fluid in a gentle and atraumatic manner enhances the recovery of morphologically and functionally competent COCs suitable for ART.

TABLE 1: Cumulus cell morphology and expansion.

Parameter	*Description*	*Impact on ART outcomes*	*Solution*
Cumulus cell layer integrity	The cumulus cell layer should appear uniform, with multiple layers of compact, healthy cells. Disruption or degeneration of these cells can indicate poor oocyte health or incomplete maturation	Degenerated or sparse cumulus cell layers are associated with poor oocyte quality, reduced developmental competence, and lower fertilization rates. The absence of cumulus cells (denuded oocytes) often indicates incomplete maturation or impaired communication between the oocyte and its microenvironment[3]	Evaluate cumulus cell morphology at the time of oocyte retrieval and before denudation. Use standardized scoring systems to assess cumulus expansion and identify oocytes with high developmental competence. Avoid mechanical stress during denudation and use enzymatic methods (e.g., hyaluronidase) at optimized concentrations and exposure times to preserve cumulus integrity[2]
Degree of cumulus expansion	Proper expansion of cumulus cells is critical for supporting oocyte maturation. Cumulus cells should exhibit multiple layers and a fluffy, loose appearance, which indicates high hyaluronic acid (HA) production and a healthy extracellular matrix	Poor cumulus expansion is often indicative of suboptimal stimulation or oocyte maturation and is linked to lower fertilization rates and impaired embryo quality. Reduced HA secretion is associated with altered expression of cumulus-specific genes (e.g., *HAS2 and PTGS2*)[4]	Optimize ovarian stimulation protocols to promote cumulus expansion. Assess cumulus cell morphology using biomarkers like *HAS2* expression or matrix metalloproteinase (MMP) activity to identify oocytes with high developmental competence. Implement regular training for embryologists to standardize the evaluation of cumulus morphology[3]

MORPHOLOGICAL ASSESSMENT OF THE OOCYTE

Morphological evaluation of the oocyte focuses on features such as ZP thickness, PV space clarity, PB integrity, and cytoplasmic texture.[1] An ideal metaphase II oocyte presents a clear, round shape with a uniformly translucent cytoplasm, a visible first PB, and a homogenous ZP of standard thickness. Aberrations in these parameters, such as vacuolations, cytoplasmic granularity, irregular zona, or fragmented polar bodies may reflect intrinsic cellular defects, metabolic imbalance, or external stressors during stimulation, retrieval, or in vitro handling. Such deviations are associated with impaired fertilization, poor cleavage, and reduced blastocyst formation **(Table 2)**. Therefore, routine morphological screening acts as a critical checkpoint for embryologists to assess developmental potential and to identify oocytes that may benefit from interventions such as assisted hatching, altered culture systems, or exclusion from intracytoplasmic sperm injection (ICSI).

GRANULARITY AND CYTOPLASMIC INCLUSIONS IN CUMULUS CELLS

Granulation or the presence of cytoplasmic inclusions within cumulus cells can be indicative of oxidative stress, exposure to environmental toxins, or metabolic imbalances **(Table 3)**. These

TABLE 2: Oocyte morphology and developmental competence correlation.

Morphological feature	*Description*	*Associated developmental competence*
Maturity (GV, MI, and MII)	GV: germinal vesicle; MI: metaphase I; MII: mature	Only MII is competent for fertilization
Zona pellucida (ZP)	*Normal:* Smooth and uniform thickness	*Abnormal ZP (thick/thin):* ↓ fertilization rate
Perivitelline space (PVS)	*Normal:* Small and clear	*Large PVS:* Associated with cytoplasmic immaturity
First polar body (PB)	Intact and appropriately sized	*Fragmented/large PB:* Possible chromosomal issues
Cytoplasm texture	Even and homogenous	*Vacuoles, granularity:* Linked to poor embryo quality
Vacuoles	None or <10 µm	*Large/multiple vacuoles:* Impaired competence
Smooth endoplasmic reticulum clusters (SERCs)	None or minimal	*SERCs:* Linked to abnormal embryo development
Ooplasm color	Light brown to transparent	*Dark ooplasm:* May indicate oxidative damage
Refractile bodies	None or small	*Large:* Associated with apoptosis, poor outcome

TABLE 3: Granularity and cytoplasmic inclusions in cumulus cells.

Parameter	*Description*	*Impact on ART outcomes*	*Solution*
Granularity of cumulus cells	Granulated or darkened cumulus cells are often a sign of metabolic stress or high ROS levels, which can impair cumulus cell function and communication with the oocyte	Granular cumulus cells are associated with reduced oocyte quality and lower fertilization potential. High ROS levels can lead to oxidative damage to both cumulus cells and the oocyte, resulting in poor embryo development[5]	Use noninvasive imaging techniques, such as DIC microscopy or fluorescence microscopy, to assess granularity. Consider supplementing culture media with antioxidants like N-acetylcysteine or melatonin to reduce ROS levels and support cumulus cell health. Minimize handling time to reduce mechanical stress and ROS generation[4]

(ART: assisted reproductive technology; DIC: differential interference contrast; ROS: reactive oxygen species)

anomalies are often associated with high levels of reactive oxygen species (ROS) and can disrupt cellular communication between the cumulus cells and the oocyte.

POLAR BODY AND PERIVITELLINE SPACE ANOMALIES

The first PB, extruded during the first meiotic division, serves as a critical marker of oocyte

TABLE 4: Polar bodies (PBs) morphology and false polar body.

Parameter	*Description*	*Impact on ART outcomes*	*Solution*
Polar body morphology	The first PB should be round, with a smooth surface and uniform cytoplasmic texture. Fragmentation or irregular PB shape indicates chromosomal segregation errors or failed cytokinesis during meiotic division	Fragmented PBs are associated with abnormal chromosomal segregation, aneuploidy, and reduced fertilization rates. Irregular PBs can complicate ICSI procedures, as they may indicate impaired cytoskeletal function[6]	Evaluate PB morphology immediately after oocyte retrieval. Use noninvasive imaging techniques to distinguish between true PB fragmentation and mechanical damage. Consider implementing meiotic spindle imaging or polar body biopsy to further assess chromosomal status when recurrent PB abnormalities are observed[3]
False PBs	False PBs are extruded cytoplasmic bodies that mimic the appearance of a true PB but lack chromosomal content. They are formed due to cytokinesis defects and can be misinterpreted during oocyte assessment	False PBs are linked to cytoskeletal dysfunction and altered gene expression during oocyte maturation. They are often associated with impaired mitochondrial activity and increased apoptosis[4]	Use high-resolution microscopy to differentiate true PBs from false PBs. Assess the cytoplasmic characteristics and positioning of the PB within the perivitelline space. Implement time-lapse imaging to monitor PB dynamics and identify abnormalities early[2]

(ART: assisted reproductive technology; ICSI: intracytoplasmic sperm injection)

maturity. Assessment of PB morphology provides valuable insights into the chromosomal status of the oocyte. Additionally, anomalies in the PV space, such as the presence of debris or inclusions, can indicate cytoplasmic or environmental stress **(Table 4)**.

PERIVITELLINE SPACE DEBRIS AND INCLUSIONS

The presence of debris or inclusions in the PV space indicates compromised oocyte health or exposure to suboptimal culture conditions. These anomalies can hinder sperm-oocyte interaction during fertilization and are frequently associated with increased oxidative stress, cytoplasmic dysregulation, or premature cortical granule exocytosis **(Table 5)**. Additionally, stimulation regimens involving supraphysiological hormone doses, particularly high levels of exogenous follicle-stimulating hormone (FSH) or luteinizing hormone (LH), and some ovulation-triggering agents, may indirectly contribute to PV debris by disrupting cytoskeletal integrity, increasing oxidative load, or altering oocyte maturation synchrony. Studies suggest that ovarian stimulation with certain gonadotropin protocols may lead to increased granulosa cell apoptosis and disrupted follicular environment, which ultimately manifests as cytoplasmic or PV abnormalities in the retrieved oocytes.[7]

CYTOPLASMIC QUALITY AND STRUCTURAL ANOMALIES

The cytoplasm of the oocyte plays a crucial role in regulating metabolic processes, supporting nuclear function, and coordinating early embryonic development. Cytoplasmic anomalies, such as vacuoles, lipid inclusions, and SERCs, can indicate compromised cellular health and reduced developmental potential **(Table 6)**.

TABLE 5: Perivitelline (PV) space debris and inclusions.

Parameter	*Description*	*Impact on ART outcomes*	*Solution*
Perivitelline space debris	PV debris consists of cellular fragments, inclusions, or other materials that accumulate between the ZP and the oocyte membrane. It often results from cytoplasmic fragmentation or environmental contamination	PV debris is associated with lower fertilization rates and impaired zygote development. Excessive PV debris can hinder sperm binding and penetration, reducing successful fertilization outcomes[2]	Use gentle handling techniques during oocyte retrieval and denudation to minimize mechanical stress. Implement regular assessments of culture media quality to identify potential sources of contamination. Use antioxidants and culture media supplements to support cytoplasmic health and reduce oxidative damage[5]

(ART: assisted reproductive technology)

TABLE 6: Cytoplasmic homogeneity and vacuoles.

Parameter	*Description*	*Impact on ART outcomes*	*Solution*
Cytoplasmic homogeneity	The cytoplasm should appear clear and homogeneous, without visible granules, inclusions, or vacuoles. Discoloration or uneven texture indicates cytoplasmic stress or metabolic dysfunction	Granular or heterogeneous cytoplasm is linked to impaired mitochondrial function, altered gene expression, and increased apoptosis. Such abnormalities are often associated with poor embryo quality and lower implantation rates[4]	Use advanced imaging techniques, such as differential interference contrast (DIC) or confocal microscopy, to evaluate cytoplasmic quality. Implement protocols to reduce oxidative stress, such as antioxidant supplementation or optimized oxygen levels (5% O_2) in culture. Consider using mitochondrial transfer or supplementation for severely compromised oocytes[3]
Vacuoles	Cytoplasmic vacuoles are clear and round inclusions that indicate cytoplasmic stress or organelle dysfunction. They may be caused by mechanical stress during handling or exposure to suboptimal culture conditions	The presence of vacuoles is associated with reduced blastocyst formation rates and an increased risk of developmental arrest. Vacuoles disrupt cytoplasmic organization and may interfere with fertilization and ICSI procedures[4]	Use noninvasive imaging techniques like time-lapse imaging to identify and monitor vacuoles during development. Consider excluding oocytes with large or multiple vacuoles from ICSI. Careful aspiration and release of ooplasm during ICSI such that sperm is not deposited in vacuoles. Optimize oocyte handling protocols to minimize mechanical stress and prevent vacuole formation[2]
Smooth endoplasmic reticulum clusters (SERCs)	SERCs are dense clusters of smooth endoplasmic reticulum observed within the oocyte cytoplasm. SERCs are linked to poor developmental potential and are associated with increased risk of implantation failure	SERCs disrupt cytoplasmic organization and mitochondrial function, leading to impaired protein synthesis, reduced ATP production, and increased risk of developmental arrest. Embryos derived from oocytes with SERCs often show poor-quality blastocysts[6]	Use high-resolution imaging techniques like confocal microscopy to detect and evaluate SERCs. Consider excluding oocytes with visible SERCs from ICSI or IVF. Review stimulation protocols and culture conditions to minimize SERC formation. Consider using time-lapse imaging to track cytoplasmic changes during oocyte maturation[3]

(ART: assisted reproductive technology; ATP: adenosine triphosphate; ICSI: intracytoplasmic sperm injection; IVF: in-vitro fertilization)

TABLE 7: Zona pellucida (ZP) thickness and homogeneity.

Parameter	*Description*	*Impact on ART outcomes*	*Solution*
Zona pellucida thickness and homogeneity	The ZP should be of uniform thickness and clarity. Uneven ZP thickness or the presence of dark zones indicates potential structural defects that may impair sperm binding and penetration	Uneven ZP thickness, extremely thin or thick zona, or the presence of dark zones may indicate structural abnormalities, which can impair sperm binding, zona penetration, or hatching. A thin or fragile ZP is more commonly observed in aged oocytes, postvitrification, or due to excessive in vitro handling. Thick zona is often noted in PCOS patients or oocytes from high gonadotropin stimulation. Structural fragility may compromise oocyte protection or embryonic expansion postfertilization[3]	For thick or uneven zona, consider mechanical zona dissection or laser-assisted hatching (LAH) prior to embryo transfer to enhance implantation potential. In fragile zona cases, minimize pipetting stress and avoid excessive hyaluronidase exposure. Ensure optimal media pH, osmolality, and avoid low-grade mineral oils that may compromise zona structure. Adhere to standardized hormone stimulation protocols to avoid over- or under-response that can affect zona morphology[4]

(ART: assisted reproductive technology; PCOS: polycystic ovarian syndrome)

ZONA PELLUCIDA STRUCTURE AND INTEGRITY

The ZP is an extracellular matrix that surrounds the oocyte, playing a crucial role in sperm binding, fertilization, and early embryonic development. Abnormalities in ZP structure or integrity can affect fertilization rates and embryo viability **(Table 7)**.

CONCLUSION

Ensuring optimal oocyte quality is fundamental for achieving success in ART. Comprehensive assessment of morphological and biochemical parameters, including cumulus cell morphology, PB integrity, cytoplasmic homogeneity, and ZP structure, provides critical insights into the developmental competence of oocytes. Identifying and troubleshooting issues such as vacuoles, lipid accumulation, PV debris, or SERCs enables embryologists to address underlying deficiencies that may compromise embryo development and implantation potential. By applying targeted strategies to mitigate these anomalies, it is possible to enhance the quality of selected oocytes and improve fertilization rates, embryo viability, and overall clinical outcomes. This holistic approach not only supports more effective embryo selection and treatment planning but also maximizes the chances of achieving successful pregnancies and healthy births for patients undergoing ART procedures.

REFERENCES

1. Alpha Scientists in Reproductive Medicine. The Istanbul consensus workshop on embryo assessment: Proceedings of an expert meeting. Reprod BioMed Online. 2011;22(6):632-46.
2. Esfandiari N, Nazemian Z. Impact of volatile organic compounds on in vitro fertilization and embryo development. J Assist Reprod Genetics. 2017;34(10):1345-54.
3. Menezo Y, Dale B. Paternal and maternal factors in preimplantation embryogenesis: Interaction

with the biochemical environment. Mol Reprod Develop. 2013;80(4):297-311.
4. Rienzi L, Ubaldi FM, Iacobelli M. Optimizing human oocyte cryopreservation: An analysis of the current state of the art. J Clin Endocrinol Metabol. 2019;104(4):1469-79.
5. Agarwal A, Gupta S, Sharma RK. Role of oxidative stress in female reproduction. Reprod Biol Endocrinol. 2016;14(1):1-21.
6. Magli MC, Van den Abbeel E, Lundin K, Royere D. Monitoring of air quality in the ART laboratory: A consensus guideline. Hum Reprod. 2016;31(7):1412-8.
7. Revelli A, Piane LD, Casano S, Molinari E, Massobrio M, Rinaudo P. Follicular fluid content and oocyte quality: from single biochemical markers to metabolomics. Reprod Biol Endocrinol. 2009;7(1):40.

SECTION

3 Fertilization and Embryo Development

CHAPTER 8

Intracytoplasmic Sperm Injection Troubleshooting

INTRODUCTION

Intracytoplasmic sperm injection (ICSI) is a sophisticated micromanipulation technique that has fundamentally transformed the landscape of assisted reproductive technology (ART), becoming the gold standard for treating severe male infertility. The procedure entails the precise injection of a single sperm directly into the cytoplasm of a mature oocyte, thus bypassing traditional barriers to fertilization, such as low sperm count, poor motility, or abnormal morphology. Although ICSI offers unparalleled control over the fertilization process, its success depends on the embryologist's expertise and the careful orchestration of multiple technical and environmental factors **(Table 1)**. Even the slightest deviation in micromanipulation technique, such as misalignment of the injection needle, variations in pipetting pressure, or exposure of gametes to nonphysiological temperatures, can result in mechanical damage to the oocyte, cytoplasmic disintegration, or failed sperm delivery, ultimately compromising fertilization rates and embryo quality **(Flowchart 1)**. Moreover, subtle changes in laboratory conditions, such as air flow, humidity, or ambient temperature, can impact oocyte viability and sperm integrity. To navigate these challenges effectively, it is essential to integrate the latest research findings and international standards such as those set by the European Society of Human Reproduction and Embryology (ESHRE), the International

TABLE 1: Environmental effects on ICSI outcomes.

Environmental factor	*Optimal condition*	*Deviation*	*Impact on ICSI outcome*
Light exposure	Dim light, filtered or red light	Bright light, UV exposure	DNA damage, zona hardening, and impaired fertilization
Temperature	36.5–37°C (stage warmer, ambient 22–25°C)	<36°C or >37°C at dish level	Spindle disruption, oocyte degeneration, and failed fertilization
Vibration	Antivibration table, minimal movement	Frequent vibration (AC and foot traffic)	Micropipette misalignment, spindle injury, and ICSI failure
Air quality	VOC-free, HEPA-filtered, and low CO_2	VOCs, dust, and CO_2 fluctuations	Oxidative stress, zona hardening, and cytoplasmic damage
Humidity	40–60% in ambient	Too low/high humidity	Media evaporation, osmotic stress on oocytes
AC/air flow	Laminar airflow, no drafts	Direct airflow on ICSI stage	Thermal shifts, media cooling, and poor micromanipulation

(HEPA: high-efficiency particulate air; ICSI: intracytoplasmic sperm injection; VOC: volatile organic compounds)

Flowchart 1: ICSI procedural stages with potential error points.

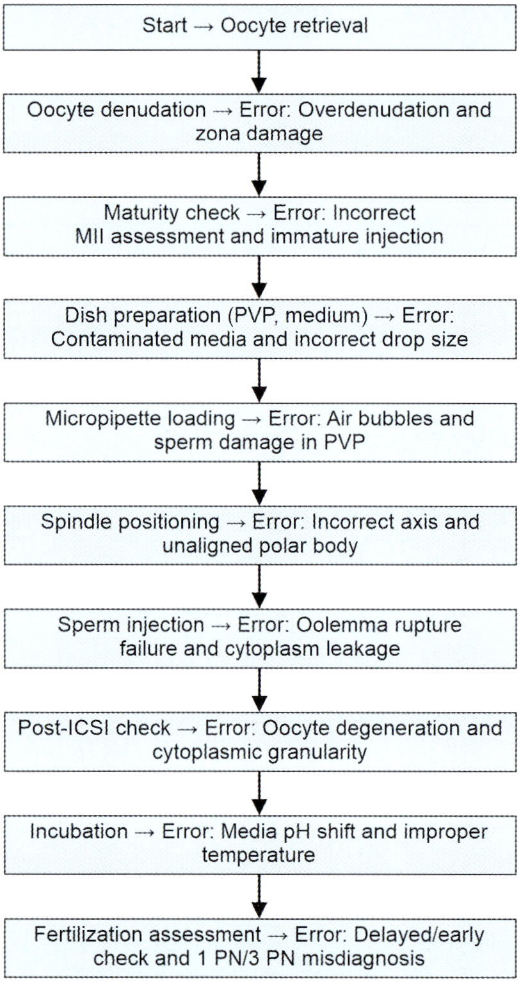

(ICSI: intracytoplasmic sperm injection; PVP: polyvinylpyrrolidone)

Organization for Standardization (ISO), and the American Society for Reproductive Medicine (ASRM). Implementing evidence-based strategies for optimizing equipment calibration, adjusting environmental parameters, and refining procedural techniques equips embryologists with the tools and knowledge to address both common and complex issues during ICSI, supporting the delivery of consistent, high-quality results and improving overall clinical outcomes for patients undergoing ART procedures.

MECHANICAL POINTS: MICROMANIPULATOR AND EQUIPMENT SETUP

Intracytoplasmic sperm injection success relies on the precise functioning and setup of the micromanipulator and associated equipment **(Table 2)**. Any mechanical malfunction or improper setup can lead to issues such as uncontrolled penetration of the oocyte, cytoplasmic damage, or failed sperm delivery.

DISH PREPARATION AND HANDLING CONDITIONS

Culture dishes and media preparation are essential aspects of ICSI that directly impact the stability and success of the procedure **(Table 3)**. Issues such as drop size, ambient temperature, and medium viscosity must be carefully managed to create an optimal environment for handling oocytes and sperm.

INTRACYTOPLASMIC SPERM INJECTION EXECUTION AND MICROMANIPULATION TECHNIQUES

The success of ICSI is heavily influenced by the precision of execution and the handling of oocytes and sperm **(Table 4)**. Issues such as misalignment, needle deflection, or repeated injections can significantly reduce fertilization rates and damage the oocyte.

CONCLUSION

Achieving successful outcomes in ICSI requires more than technical proficiency; it demands a comprehensive understanding of the intricate interplay between micromanipulation

TABLE 2: Troubleshooting micromanipulation and ICSI workstation parameters.

Issue	*Description*	*Impact on ART outcomes*	*Solution*
Vibrations during ICSI	Vibrations at the ICSI workstation can result from external sources like AC units, nearby laboratory equipment, or structural instability. They may also arise from subtle internal factors such as elbow contact with the table, foot pressure on unstable floors, trolleys, swinging doors, or footwear lacking cushioning. Even air currents from vents or open doors can destabilize the micromanipulation setup, compromising injection precision and oocyte integrity	Vibrations result in needle misalignment, oocyte displacement, and difficulty in precisely penetrating the oocyte, leading to mechanical damage or poor sperm deposition	Use antivibration tables as recommended by ISO standards. Isolate the workstation from vibration sources. Ensure that the ICSI workstation is not positioned near AC vents or high-traffic areas. Perform regular vibration checks and adjust workstation placement if necessary[1]
Pressure controls and microinjector settings	Inconsistent pressure settings in microinjectors can cause sudden or jerky movements of the injection or holding pipette, compromising precision. This may be worsened by improper insertion or loose tightening of micropipettes, poor meniscus monitoring in PVP or culture drops, or unrecognized air bubbles in the system. If not addressed, these factors can lead to sudden fluid ejection, floating of oocytes, or dislodgment during manipulation	Uncontrolled penetration of the oocyte, damage to the zona pellucida, or cytoplasmic leakage can result from improper pressure controls	Follow standard operating procedures (SOPs) for microinjector calibration before each session. Adjust positive and negative pressure settings based on sample requirements. Implement regular equipment maintenance and follow ISO 20387 standards for laboratory calibration and validation[2]
Toolholder and needle alignment	Misalignment of the injection needle and holding pipette in the toolholder, causing deflection during micromanipulation	Misalignment causes skewed needle entry angles, cytoplasmic damage, or difficulty in stabilizing the oocyte during injection	Follow ISO 15189 recommendations for regular alignment checks of micromanipulation tools. Alignment of micropipettes to be done on lower most magnification and confirmed on higher magnification for fine adjustments. Ensure that the needle and holding pipette are parallel and at the correct angle. Perform routine validation of microscope and toolholder alignment using calibration markers and mock samples[3]

Contd...

Contd...

Issue	*Description*	*Impact on ART outcomes*	*Solution*
Axis and fine control issues	Improper calibration of the micromanipulator's X, Y, and Z-axis controls results in unwanted movements and makes it difficult to achieve smooth and precise manipulation	Unwanted axis movements can cause damage to the oocyte, misalignment of the needle, and poor sperm deposition	Calibrate X, Y, and Z axes regularly. Test fine controls on inert samples to ensure precision before handling oocytes. Adjust axis sensitivity settings based on sample properties and laboratory conditions[4]
Light intensity and microscope settings	High-intensity light exposure leads to phototoxic damage, while low-intensity light makes it difficult to visualize the procedure	Photodamage can impair oocyte quality and reduce fertilization rates, while poor visibility increases the risk of mechanical damage during micromanipulation	Use the lowest effective light intensity according to ICSI guidelines. Adjust microscope settings to enhance contrast and resolution. Consider using polarized light or DIC microscopy to improve visualization without increasing light exposure[5]

(ART: assisted reproductive technology; DIC: differential interference contrast; ICSI: intracytoplasmic sperm injection; ISO: International Organization for Standardization; PVP: polyvinylpyrrolidone)

TABLE 3: Troubleshooting ICSI dish preparation and pipetting challenges.

Issue	*Description*	*Impact on ART outcomes*	*Solution*
Large drops mixing in dish	Large drops of culture media can merge during handling, altering ionic concentration and buffer stability, thereby disrupting the delicate microenvironment essential for gamete or embryo viability. Drops should be placed close enough for efficient workflow but sufficiently spaced to avoid unintentional mixing. Position them within the central field of view under the microscope; placing drops too far apart or outside the visual plane can increase the risk of losing track of gametes or accidentally dragging media during pipetting	Changes in pH, osmolarity, or ion concentration can negatively affect oocyte and sperm function	Use smaller microdrops (10–20 µL) overlaid with oil to prevent mixing and evaporation, as recommended by the WHO and ESHRE guidelines. Distribute the drops in a symmetrical layout that allows easy movement of the micropipette between injection, wash, and holding areas while maintaining visibility within the microscope's field. Ensure each drop has uniform volume to avoid concentration variability, and place wash drops in accessible positions near the center of the dish for efficient rinsing during pipetting. Equilibrate the dish at 37°C with a pH range of 7.2–7.4 to create a physiologically stable and consistent microenvironment[6]

Contd...

Contd...

Issue	*Description*	*Impact on ART outcomes*	*Solution*
Ambient temperature and airflow control	Variations in temperature or direct airflow from AC units cause rapid changes in culture media temperature	Temperature fluctuations lead to thermal shock, affecting oocyte and sperm viability	Maintain a controlled laboratory environment at 37°C and minimize airflow, following ISO 14644 standards for cleanroom environments. Use enclosed workstations with heating stages and perform ICSI under an oil overlay to ensure thermal stability. Minimize exposure of open drops to ambient conditions[2]
Viscous samples and sticky cytoplasm	High viscosity of the cytoplasm or medium complicates the injection process, making it difficult to deposit the sperm properly	Increased viscosity can lead to resistance during injection, causing cytoplasmic damage or improper sperm placement	Adjust the injection speed and pressure to accommodate changes in media viscosity, ensuring smooth penetration of the oolemma and minimizing cellular trauma. Use polyvinylpyrrolidone (PVP) solutions of appropriate viscosity to reduce sperm motility for better control during injection and precondition the injection pipette in the PVP drop to reduce surface tension variability. In cases involving poor-quality or partially motile sperm, modified ICSI approaches may be employed. Follow ESHRE guidelines and laboratory-specific protocols to ensure that any alterations to the standard ICSI technique maintain the physiological integrity of both gametes and maximize fertilization outcomes[7]
Partially denuded oocytes	Oocytes that are not completely denuded may retain cumulus or corona radiata cells, making it difficult to visualize the polar body and zona pellucida during ICSI	Residual cells can obstruct needle entry and increase the risk of oocyte damage	Ensure complete denudation using enzymatic and mechanical methods. Use hyaluronidase at 40–80 IU/mL and gentle mechanical pipetting. Check for residual cells under a microscope and remove them using a fine capillary pipette[3]
Sticky micropipette or holding pipette carrying sperm to oocyte	Accumulation of PVP or other sticky substances on the micropipette causes sperm to adhere to the pipette, making it difficult to release the sperm into the oocyte	Failed sperm injection attempts, increased handling time, and potential damage to the oocyte	Precondition the injection pipette in a PVP drop to reduce sticking. Rinse the pipette in a clean medium drop before and after each injection to prevent PVP build-up. Adjust pipette pressure settings to facilitate smooth sperm release[7]

(ART: assisted reproductive technology; ESHRE: European Society of Human Reproduction and Embryology; ICSI: intracytoplasmic sperm injection; ISO: International Organization for Standardization; WHO: World Health Organization)

TABLE 4: Troubleshooting in micromanipulation techniques.

Issue	*Description*	*Impact on ART outcomes*	*Solution*
Axis and injection needle alignment issues	Misalignment of the injection needle and the holding pipette can result in skewed entry angles and increased resistance during injection	Misalignment damages the zona pellucida, causes cytoplasmic leakage, or results in failed sperm delivery	Align the needle and pipette parallel to each other and at the correct angle. Use precise focusing capabilities to ensure proper alignment. Follow ESHRE and ASRM recommendations for micromanipulator alignment and calibration to achieve optimal needle positioning[1]
Repeat ICSI on multiple oocytes	Repeated ICSI attempts on multiple oocytes can lead to increased handling time, media exposure, and potential oocyte damage	Prolonged exposure to nonphysiological conditions can impair oocyte quality and reduce fertilization rates	Minimize the number of oocytes handled simultaneously. Prepare individual dishes for each oocyte if necessary, and complete injection within a 5-minute window. Use a temperature-controlled stage and validated equipment to maintain environmental stability[3]
Holding pipette in PVP carrying sperm to oocyte	Holding pipette with sperm in PVP solution can cause sperm to adhere to the pipette or disrupt the injection process	Difficulties in sperm release, improper sperm placement, and increased handling time	Precondition the pipette in a PVP drop and rinse in a clean medium drop before sperm handling. Use a low-viscosity medium to facilitate sperm release and follow ISO guidelines for preconditioning pipettes[7]

(ART: assisted reproductive technology; ASRM: American Society for Reproductive Medicine; ESHRE: European Society of Human Reproduction and Embryology; ICSI: intracytoplasmic sperm injection; ISO: International Organization for Standardization; PVP: polyvinylpyrrolidone)

techniques, equipment precision, and the biological sensitivities of oocytes and sperm. This chapter has outlined the multitude of factors influencing ICSI performance, offering a practical troubleshooting guide to mechanical issues, environmental stressors, and procedural inconsistencies. Vibrations from the laboratory floor, elbow rests, trolley wheels, poorly secured doors, footwear movement, or turbulent air currents can transfer subtle mechanical disruptions to the workstation, compromising stability. Misaligned micromanipulators, abrupt pressure shifts in microinjectors, improper pipette insertion, poorly tightened screws, or failure to monitor the meniscus of media and polyvinylpyrrolidone (PVP) can result in erratic movement, bubbles, or even oocyte displacement during injection. Large media drops placed too far apart or beyond the focal plane of the microscope can merge, altering osmolarity or disrupting the microenvironment. Furthermore, biological challenges such as fragile oocyte zona, sticky cytoplasm, or partially denuded oocytes can impede the smooth execution of the injection, increasing the likelihood of oocyte trauma or suboptimal fertilization. All of these issues highlight the importance of not only refined motor skills but also close attention to detail, calibration, environmental control, and synchronized teamwork. Looking forward, advances in automated micromanipulation platforms, robotics, real-time feedback control systems, and artificial intelligence-assisted software are poised to standardize the injection process, minimize variability, and enhance precision. By bridging current manual limitations and preparing for emerging innovations, embryologists can transform ICSI from a technically demanding procedure into a more streamlined, reliable, and success-driven component of assisted reproduction.

REFERENCES

1. Vanderzwalmen P, Zech H, Vanderzwalmen S. Cryopreservation of in vitro matured oocytes. Reprod BioMed Online. 2016;33(1):11-24.
2. Nagy ZP, Varghese AC, Agarwal A. Practical Manual of In Vitro Fertilization: Advanced Methods and Novel Devices. Germany: Springer; 2018.
3. Rienzi L, Ubaldi FM, Iacobelli M. Optimizing human oocyte cryopreservation: An analysis of the current state of the art. J Clin Endocrinol Metabol. 2019;104(4):1469-79.
4. Wang X, Liu Y, Zheng Y. The influence of the microenvironment on ICSI success rates: A review of laboratory protocols and equipment calibration. Fertil Steril. 2021;116(4):882-9.
5. Parmegiani L, Cognigni GE, Bernardi S, Troilo E, Maccarini G. Comparison of two hyaluronidase preparations in denuding cumulus-oocyte complexes for intracytoplasmic sperm injection: Evaluation of denudation time, oocyte morphology, and embryo quality. J Assist Reprod Genetics. 2014;31(4):463-9.
6. Agarwal A, Gupta S, Sharma R. Andrological Evaluation of Male Infertility: A Laboratory Guide. Germany: Springer; 2016.
7. Palermo G, Joris H, Devroey P, Van Steirteghem AC. Intracytoplasmic Sperm Injection: State of the Art in Humans. Reprod BioMed Online. 2017;36(6):747-62.

CHAPTER

9 Fertilization Assessment

INTRODUCTION

Fertilization assessment is a pivotal component of assisted reproductive technology (ART), offering critical insights into the success of the fertilization process and the developmental potential of embryos. Through careful evaluation of fertilization patterns such as the formation and structure of pronuclei, cytoplasmic changes, and key biochemical indicators, embryologists can identify high quality embryos and detect underlying issues that may hinder developmental progression **(Table 1)**. During this stage, the zygote is formed as a single cell containing the complete diploid genome derived from both the egg and the sperm. The zygote is distinct from the embryo, which refers to the multicellular structure that forms following the first mitotic division. In several countries, this distinction has ethical and legal implications, as the zygote may not yet be considered an embryo for regulatory or legislative purposes. This impacts decisions regarding storage, manipulation, and clinical use. Accurate assessment of parameters such as pronuclear symmetry, the number and placement of nucleolar precursor bodies, and the appearance of the cytoplasm provides valuable information regarding chromosomal status and cell health. Additional evaluation of mitochondrial activity, cellular redox potential, and the distribution of cortical granules further enhances the ability to predict successful fertilization and embryo development.

UNDERSTANDING NORMAL FERTILIZATION PATTERNS AND CRITERIA

Understanding normal fertilization patterns is essential in assessing the developmental

TABLE 1: Fertilization timing checkpoints.

Timepoint	*Definition*	*Optimal timing (Post-ICSI)*	*Clinical significance*
t_0	Time of ICSI (sperm injection)	0 hours	Reference time for embryo development timeline
tPNF	Time of pronuclear formation	6–8 hours post-ICSI	Indicator of normal fertilization initiation
t_2PN	Time of 2 pronuclei visible	16–18 hours post-ICSI	Confirms normal fertilization; 2PN1PB is ideal
t_2	Time of first cleavage (2-cell stage)	24–27 hours post-ICSI	Early cleavage linked to higher implantation potential

(ICSI: intracytoplasmic sperm injection)

TABLE 2: Zygote Z-score grading scheme (based on Scott et al.).

Grade	*Pronuclei (PN) position*	*Nucleolar precursor bodies (NPBs)*	*Cytoplasm*	*Clinical implication*
Z1	Centrally located, adjacent	Symmetrical, equal number in each PN	Clear and homogeneous	High implantation and blastocyst potential
Z2	Slightly off-center	Unequal NPB number	Mild granularity	Moderate developmental potential
Z3	Eccentric PN position	Scattered or clumped NPBs	Cytoplasmic granules	Low potential and monitor closely
Z4	PN far apart, abnormal size	Irregular or no NPBs	Dark or vacuolated	Poor prognosis; usually nonviable

potential of embryos and optimizing clinical outcomes in ART **(Table 2)**. Key morphological and cellular indicators such as pronuclear formation, nucleolar precursor body (NPB) distribution, cytoplasmic appearance, and cortical integrity serve as predictive markers of zygotic health **(Table 3)**. Evaluating these parameters allows embryologists to distinguish between normal and aberrant fertilization events, guiding embryo selection and identifying procedural or biological issues that may compromise success.

ASSESSING ABNORMAL FERTILIZATION PATTERNS AND THEIR IMPLICATIONS

Assessing abnormal fertilization patterns is crucial for identifying failures in gamete function, oocyte activation, and fertilization mechanisms during ART **(Table 4)**. Deviations such as tripronuclear zygotes (3PN), single pronucleus (1PN), or disrupted pronuclear morphology often reflect chromosomal misalignments, parthenogenetic activation, or mechanical errors during ICSI. These abnormalities compromise embryo viability, leading to developmental arrest or aneuploidy **(Flowchart 1)**. Recognizing these patterns allows embryologists to refine laboratory protocols, optimize gamete handling, and implement preventive strategies to enhance fertilization outcomes and clinical success.

BIOCHEMICAL AND GENETIC INDICATORS OF FERTILIZATION QUALITY

Understanding the biochemical and genetic indicators of fertilization quality is crucial in predicting embryonic developmental potential and optimizing outcomes in ART **(Table 5)**. While morphological evaluation remains fundamental, cellular processes such as redox balance, mitochondrial function, and cortical granule distribution offer deeper insights into the molecular health of the oocyte and zygote. Disruptions in these processes, whether due to oxidative stress, impaired mitochondrial activity, or abnormal NPB patterns can compromise fertilization, genome activation, and subsequent embryo viability. Incorporating biochemical assessments alongside traditional observations enables embryologists to more accurately identify viable embryos and adopt corrective strategies when deviations are observed, thereby refining the ART workflow and improving clinical success rates.

TABLE 3: Key morphological and functional parameters in pronuclear and zygote assessment for optimizing ART outcomes.

Parameter	*Description*	*Impact on ART outcomes*	*Solution*
Pronuclear (PN) formation	Formation of two distinct pronuclei (2PN) in the oocyte cytoplasm. Pronuclei should be similar in size, with well-defined boundaries and centrally positioned. Symmetrical formation indicates successful fertilization[1]	Symmetrical 2PN formation with even NPB distribution suggests balanced parental genomic contribution and high developmental potential. Abnormal PN morphology reduces embryo quality	Evaluate 2PN formation 16–18 hours postinsemination or ICSI. Use time-lapse imaging to track pronuclear dynamics. Review sperm preparation and ICSI techniques if abnormalities are frequent[2]
Symmetry of pronuclei	Both pronuclei should be of equal size, with no evidence of fragmentation or vacuolation. Symmetry reflects proper chromosomal alignment and zygotic genome activation	Symmetrical pronuclei are associated with high-quality embryos and reduced risk of aneuploidy	Perform regular training and calibration for embryologists on pronuclear morphology assessment. Use standardized criteria and imaging modalities for consistency
Number and distribution of nucleolar precursor bodies (NPBs)	NPBs should be evenly distributed within each pronucleus, with uniform size and shape. NPBs are markers of transcriptional activity and zygotic genome activation	Abnormal NPB distribution indicates poor transcriptional activity and may signal developmental arrest or chromosomal anomalies	Use scoring systems such as Z-score to evaluate NPB distribution. Implement time-lapse monitoring to analyze NPB dynamics and identify early signs of developmental issues[3]
Cytoplasmic appearance	Cytoplasm should be homogeneous, without vacuoles or granulation, and with a regular texture indicative of proper organelle distribution	Abnormal cytoplasmic appearance (e.g., granular or vacuolated) is linked to poor oocyte quality and lower fertilization potential	Use confocal or DIC microscopy to evaluate cytoplasmic quality. Optimize culture conditions and use antioxidant-enriched media to support cytoplasmic health[4]
Cortical zone integrity	Thickness and uniformity of the cortical zone affect the fertilization process and the oocyte's response to sperm entry. Proper cortical reaction prevents polyspermy and ensures successful fertilization	Abnormal cortical zone thickness or premature granule exocytosis can lead to polyspermy or failed fertilization, reducing developmental potential	Optimize oocyte handling and timing of ICSI. Use calcium ionophores or media supplements to support cortical zone integrity. Assess cortical granule distribution using confocal microscopy[5]

(ART: assisted reproductive technology; DIC: differential interference contrast; ICSI: intracytoplasmic sperm injection)

TABLE 4: Abnormal fertilization patterns: descriptions, clinical impact, and corrective strategies in ART.

Abnormal fertilization pattern	*Description*	*Impact on ART outcomes*	*Solution*
Tripronuclear with one polar body (3PN1PB)	Presence of three pronuclei (3PN) and one polar body (1PB) due to polyspermy or parthenogenesis	3PN oocytes are nonviable for embryonic development and are excluded from further culture. Indicates compromised fertilization mechanisms and reduced gamete quality	Review sperm concentration during insemination to prevent polyspermy. Adjust zona hardening protocols, such as exposure to calcium ionophores, to enhance the zona reaction[6]
Single pronucleus with three polar bodies (1PN3PB)	Presence of a single pronucleus with three polar bodies due to meiotic errors or parthenogenetic activation	High likelihood of chromosomal abnormalities. Such zygotes are nonviable and unsuitable for embryo culture	Investigate potential causes of meiotic spindle disruption (e.g., exposure to toxins or mechanical damage). Optimize oocyte retrieval timing and ICSI techniques to avoid spindle damage
Abnormal pronuclear size and NPB distribution	Pronuclei with disproportionate sizes or uneven distribution of NPBs suggest chromosomal misalignment or failed zygotic genome activation	Lower developmental potential and increased risk of aneuploidy	Use advanced imaging techniques (e.g., confocal microscopy) to assess pronuclear size and NPB distribution. Implement genetic screening or preimplantation genetic testing (PGT) if recurrent abnormalities are observed[2]
Polyspermy (Multiple pronuclei)	Fertilization by more than one sperm, leading to more than two pronuclei (e.g., 3PN and 4PN)	Polyspermic zygotes are nonviable and are typically discarded. Indicates compromised zona pellucida integrity or failed cortical reaction	Optimize sperm concentration and incubation time during insemination to reduce polyspermy risk. Consider zona hardening agents such as calcium ionophore or zona pellucida thickness modification techniques[5]
Single pronucleus (1PN)	Formation of a single pronucleus due to parthenogenetic activation, failed pronuclear fusion, or abnormal oocyte activation	Single pronuclear zygotes have a high probability of chromosomal abnormalities and are unsuitable for embryo culture	Review oocyte activation protocols and consider adjusting ICSI parameters (e.g., sperm injection speed and depth) to promote proper male and female pronuclear formation[3]

(ART: assisted reproductive technology; ICSI: intracytoplasmic sperm injection; NPB: nucleolar precursor body)

Flowchart 1: Normal versus abnormal fertilization—causes and follow-up steps.

Fertilization check (16–18 hours post-ICSI) → Evaluate pronuclei and polar bodies

↓

Is fertilization normal? (2PN + 1PB)
├ Yes → Proceed to culture → Cleavage monitoring
└ No

↓

Abnormal fertilization detected:
├ 1PN → Cause: Asynchronous PN formation and parthenogenesis
├ 3PN → Cause: Polyspermy and oocyte activation error
├ 0PN → Cause: Failed activation and sperm decondensation failure

↓

Follow-up:
- Discard 3PN or abnormal embryos (nonviable)
- Consider ICSI protocol review, sperm quality assessment
- Possible zona hardening? → Evaluate denudation and enzyme use

(ICSI: intracytoplasmic sperm injection; PN: pronucleus)

TABLE 5: Biochemical markers of oocyte quality and their impact on ART outcomes.

Biochemical indicator	*Description*	*Impact on ART outcomes*	*Solution*
Redox potential and oxidative stress	Balance between oxidative and reductive processes within the oocyte, indicative of cellular health. Elevated redox potential suggests oxidative stress, leading to DNA damage and impaired function	High redox potential is associated with reduced fertilization rates and increased oocyte degeneration	Measure redox status using specific dyes or markers (e.g., roGFP). Supplement culture media with antioxidants like melatonin or N-acetylcysteine to reduce oxidative damage[7]
Mitochondrial function and mutations	Mitochondria provide energy for zygotic division and development. Mitochondrial mutations or dysfunction impair ATP production and increase the risk of developmental arrest and aneuploidy	Mitochondrial abnormalities reduce fertilization potential and embryo viability, often leading to failed implantation or pregnancy loss	Assess mitochondrial function using fluorescent markers or mtDNA copy number analysis. Consider mitochondrial supplementation or replacement strategies to enhance oocyte quality[8]
Cortical granule distribution and zona reaction	Cortical granules play a key role in the zona reaction, preventing polyspermy. Abnormal distribution or premature exocytosis can compromise the zona reaction, allowing multiple sperm penetration	Inadequate cortical reaction leads to polyspermy or failed fertilization, decreasing developmental potential and embryo quality	Evaluate cortical granule distribution using confocal microscopy. Optimize oocyte handling and timing of ICSI to prevent premature granule exocytosis. Use calcium ionophore treatment to regulate cortical granule release[5]

Contd...

Contd...

Biochemical indicator	*Description*	*Impact on ART outcomes*	*Solution*
Nucleolar precursor body (NPB) distribution	NPBs indicate transcriptional activity within the pronuclei. Uniform size and even distribution are signs of proper zygotic genome activation and balanced chromosomal alignment	Abnormal NPB patterns are associated with developmental arrest and lower implantation potential	Use scoring systems such as the Z-score to evaluate NPB distribution. Monitor pronuclear morphology and NPB dynamics using time-lapse imaging or confocal microscopy[5]
Cytoplasmic texture and organelle distribution	Homogeneous cytoplasm indicates balanced organelle distribution and healthy metabolic activity. Granular or vacuolated cytoplasm may reflect oxidative damage, abnormal organelle function, or altered metabolism	Granular or vacuolated cytoplasm is linked to poor fertilization rates, lower embryo quality, and increased risk of chromosomal abnormalities	Evaluate cytoplasmic appearance using advanced imaging modalities (e.g., DIC or confocal microscopy). Implement cytoplasmic quality enhancement strategies, such as optimizing culture conditions and supplementing media with mitochondria-targeted agents[4]

(ART: assisted reproductive technology; DIC: differential interference contrast; ICSI: intracytoplasmic sperm injection)

FERTILIZATION GRADING AND SELECTION CRITERIA

Fertilization grading plays a critical role in selecting embryos with the highest developmental potential in ART. By evaluating specific criteria such as pronuclear symmetry, polar body number, nucleolar precursor body distribution, and cytoplasmic clarity, embryologists can distinguish between normally and abnormally fertilized oocytes **(Table 6)**. Normal fertilization patterns are closely linked with successful implantation and pregnancy outcomes, while abnormal patterns may signal chromosomal instability or fertilization failure.[1] Establishing clear selection benchmarks using standardized grading systems helps to ensure the identification of viable embryos for transfer or cryopreservation, ultimately optimizing clinical results and reducing the risk of failed cycles.

CONCLUSION

Understanding the nuances of fertilization is a critical step in optimizing outcomes in ART. By thoroughly assessing pronuclear formation, cytoplasmic dynamics, and various biochemical markers, embryologists can gain valuable insights into the health and developmental potential of embryos. Each fertilization pattern, whether normal or abnormal, provides clues about the underlying quality of the gametes and the conditions of the fertilization process. For instance, abnormalities like tripronuclear (3PN) formation or the presence of a single pronucleus (1PN) can highlight potential issues with chromosomal alignment, oocyte activation, or procedural errors. Evaluating factors such as mitochondrial health, oxidative stress levels, and cortical granule distribution further deepens our understanding of how these biological components interact to

TABLE 6: Criteria for normal versus abnormal fertilization and their implications in ART outcomes.

Criteria	*Description*	*Impact on ART outcomes*	*Solution*
Normal fertilization criteria	Normal fertilization is characterized by two symmetrical pronuclei, each with evenly distributed NPBs, and two polar bodies. Cytoplasm should appear clear and homogeneous, without vacuoles or granulation	Zygotes with normal fertilization patterns have higher implantation and pregnancy rates	Use standardized grading systems and international guidelines (e.g., ESHRE and ASRM) to assess zygote quality. Implement time-lapse imaging to track fertilization dynamics and ensure accurate assessment[2]
Abnormal fertilization criteria	Abnormal fertilization includes the presence of more than two pronuclei, single pronucleus, fragmented pronuclei, or uneven cytoplasmic texture. Such patterns are indicative of chromosomal imbalances or meiotic errors	Abnormal zygotes have a lower potential for embryo development and increased risk of genetic anomalies	Exclude abnormal zygotes from embryo culture. Consider advanced diagnostic techniques such as preimplantation genetic testing (PGT) to identify potential chromosomal abnormalities. Optimize laboratory protocols to minimize mechanical or environmental factors contributing to abnormal fertilization[6]

(ART: assisted reproductive technology; ASRM: American Society for Reproductive Medicine; ESHRE: European Society of Human Reproduction and Embryology; NPB: nucleolar precursor body)

shape embryo quality. When these assessments are performed with precision and supported by advanced technologies like time-lapse imaging and biochemical assays, embryologists are better equipped to make informed decisions on embryo selection and treatment modifications.

REFERENCES

1. Sathananthan AH, Trounson AO. Fertilization and early human development in assisted reproduction. Reprod BioMed Online. 2013;26(3):311-24.
2. Alpha Scientists in Reproductive Medicine. The Istanbul Consensus Workshop on embryo assessment: Proceedings of an expert meeting. Reprod BioMed Online. 2011;22(6):632-46.
3. Tesarik J, Greco E, Rienzi L. The predictive value of pronuclear morphology and dynamics for embryo development and implantation. J Assist Reprod Genetics. 2015;32(10):1435-41.
4. Rienzi L, Ubaldi FM, Iacobelli M. Optimizing human oocyte cryopreservation: An analysis of the current state of the art. J Clin Endocrinol Metabol. 2019;104(4):1469-79.
5. Abbott AL, Fissore RA, Ducibella T. The role of cortical granules in fertilization and polyspermy prevention. J Reprod Immunol. 2015;108:1-7.
6. De Rycke M, Bergh C, Mertes H. Biopsy-related risks for human embryo and fetus: Time to change the focus. Hum Reprod Update. 2020;26(4):470-92.
7. Bentov Y, Casper RF. The aging oocyte—can mitochondrial function be improved? Fertil Steril. 2014;99(1):18-22.
8. Wai T, Ao A, Zhang X, Pinto M. The role of mitochondrial mutations in male infertility. Hum Reprod Update. 2010;16(2):143-58.

CHAPTER

10 Embryo Assessment

INTRODUCTION

Embryo assessment is a cornerstone of assisted reproductive technology (ART), providing crucial insights into the developmental competence and implantation potential of embryos. Evaluations at the cleavage stage (Day 3) and blastocyst stage (Day 5) are standard practice, where morphological markers such as blastomere number, symmetry, degree of fragmentation, multinucleation, and compaction are closely examined. Advanced assessments go beyond morphology and include time-lapse imaging, which captures dynamic parameters like cleavage timing and synchrony of divisions, offering a more nuanced prediction of embryo viability. Additionally, metabolic profiling of spent culture media evaluates the embryo's nutrient consumption and by-product secretion, giving indirect but valuable cues about mitochondrial activity and cellular function. Biochemical indicators, such as mitochondrial distribution, ATP content, and oxidative stress markers, can further elucidate embryo health, while molecular markers like gene expression profiles and epigenetic status are being explored to refine embryo selection. Techniques such as preimplantation genetic testing (PGT) are employed to screen for aneuploidies and single-gene disorders, especially in patients with recurrent implantation failure or advanced maternal age, enhancing the precision of embryo transfer decisions. Together, the integration of morphological, kinetic, metabolic, and genetic criteria allows for a comprehensive, evidence-based approach to embryo assessment, ultimately maximizing clinical success and offering a more personalized ART strategy tailored to the patient's reproductive profile.

STAGES OF EMBRYO DEVELOPMENT AND KEY ASSESSMENT PARAMETERS

Embryo evaluation is conducted at different developmental stages, each presenting unique morphological and biochemical markers that are indicative of the embryo's health and viability. Detailed assessment at these stages helps to identify embryos with optimal developmental potential **(Tables 1 and 2)**.

COMMON ISSUES DURING EMBRYO DEVELOPMENT AND THEIR IMPLICATIONS

Developmental issues, such as fragmentation, asymmetrical division, degeneration, and sudden arrest, can hinder embryo quality and viability **(Table 3)**. Understanding these issues and their causes is essential for identifying embryos with the best developmental potential and implementing corrective measures **(Fig. 1)**.

BIOCHEMICAL AND GENETIC FACTORS IN EMBRYO DEVELOPMENT

Embryo development is regulated by complex biochemical and genetic interactions that dictate cell division, differentiation, and viability

TABLE 1: Cleavage stage embryo assessment.

Parameter	*Description*	*Impact on ART outcomes*	*Solution*
Blastomere number and symmetry	A good-quality Day 3 embryo typically has 6–8 blastomeres of equal size and shape, indicating proper cleavage and division. Asymmetry or uneven blastomere sizes can suggest chromosomal abnormalities or compromised cell division machinery	Symmetrical blastomeres are associated with higher implantation and live birth rates, as they indicate balanced chromosomal segregation and healthy cytoskeletal organization. Unequal or asymmetrical blastomeres suggest aneuploidy, mitochondrial dysfunction, or other genetic defects	Ensure that culture conditions, such as stable temperature and pH, are optimized to support synchronized blastomere division. Minimize mechanical stress during handling to avoid disrupting spindle formation and cleavage patterns. Conduct genetic testing, such as preimplantation genetic testing for aneuploidy (PGT-A), if asymmetry is frequent[1]
Percentage and localization of fragmentation	Fragmentation refers to anucleate cytoplasmic fragments within embryos, often due to apoptosis or abnormal division. Large coarse fragments typically reflect more severe cellular damage, while small, granulated ones may suggest milder stress. Fragment pattern and distribution; whether central or peripheral can impact development, with >25% fragmentation linked to poorer outcomes	High fragmentation levels (>25%) reduce embryo viability, hinder blastomere communication, and increase the likelihood of implantation failure. The localization of fragments can influence blastomere communication and signal potential stress or damage within the embryo	Optimize culture media with antiapoptotic agents such as hyaluronan or low oxygen (5%) culture conditions to minimize apoptosis-induced fragmentation. Use time-lapse imaging to distinguish reversible versus irreversible fragmentation. Consider early transfer or vitrification of embryos with moderate fragmentation levels (<25%) if they show good cleavage patterns[2]
Blastomere degeneration	Blastomere degeneration is marked by dark, vacuolated, or fragmented blastomeres due to factors such as oxidative stress, impaired mitochondrial activity, or poor culture conditions. Pale blastomeres, especially when located peripherally, may indicate cytoplasmic dilution or suboptimal metabolic function. These degenerative signs reflect reduced developmental potential and may warrant exclusion from transfer consideration	Degenerated blastomeres indicate cellular damage and metabolic dysfunction, lowering overall embryo quality and reducing the likelihood of forming a viable blastocyst. Degeneration is often linked to mitochondrial mutations, failed DNA repair mechanisms, or high oxidative stress	Reduce oxidative stress in culture media by adding antioxidants like melatonin or glutathione. Regularly monitor culture medium quality, pH, and osmolarity. Ensure that all culture components, including oil overlays and incubators, are equilibrated properly. Use biomarkers like mitochondrial membrane potential (MMP) or reactive oxygen species (ROS) assays to assess embryo health and identify those at risk of degeneration[3]

Contd...

Contd...

Parameter	*Description*	*Impact on ART outcomes*	*Solution*
Asynchronous cleavage	Asynchronous cleavage refers to uneven or uncoordinated blastomere division, often leading to odd cell numbers like 5 or 9. This may reflect disrupted cell cycle regulation or chromosomal issues. Unequal blastomere size, abnormal orientation, and inconsistent measurement across cells can further indicate poor embryo quality and reduced implantation potential	Asynchronous division is indicative of compromised chromosomal integrity, spindle misalignment, or cytoskeletal disorganization. It is associated with reduced blastocyst formation rates and poor developmental potential	Monitor cleavage patterns using time-lapse imaging to identify embryos with abnormal division patterns. Adjust culture conditions to support synchronized division, such as using media with growth factors like IGF or LIF. Conduct spindle checkpoint analysis to evaluate cell-cycle progression in embryos with frequent asynchronous divisions[4]
Cellular and cytoplasmic quality	The presence of vacuoles, dark inclusions, or granular cytoplasm in blastomeres suggests cytoplasmic stress, impaired organelle function, or suboptimal environmental exposure. Additionally, the appearance of multiple nuclei within a single blastomere (multinucleation) or visible nucleoli indicates aberrant cell division, which is often linked to chromosomal abnormalities and reduced developmental competence[5]	Poor cytoplasmic quality is linked to mitochondrial dysfunction, reduced ATP production, and impaired cellular metabolism, all of which lower implantation potential and embryo viability	Use high-resolution imaging as differential interference contrast (DIC) to evaluate cytoplasmic quality. Minimize mechanical and thermal stress during oocyte retrieval, sperm injection, and embryo culture. Implement quality control measures for culture medium to ensure stable pH, osmolarity, and temperature[3]

(ART: assisted reproductive technology; IGF: insulin-like growth factor; LIF: leukemia inhibitory factor)

TABLE 2: Blastocyst stage embryo assessment.

Parameter	*Description*	*Impact on ART outcomes*	*Solution*
Blastocyst expansion and hatching	A good-quality blastocyst should show full expansion with a well-defined inner cell mass (ICM) and trophectoderm (TE) layer. Hatching or hatched blastocysts have the highest implantation potential due to successful zona thinning and expansion	Fully expanded and hatched blastocysts are associated with the highest implantation and live birth rates. Incomplete expansion or premature hatching may indicate developmental arrest or compromised energy metabolism within the blastocyst	Optimize culture conditions, including controlled gas concentrations (5–6% CO_2 and 5% O_2) and stable temperature (37°C), to support blastocyst expansion and hatching. Implement time-lapse monitoring to track blastocyst expansion dynamics and identify embryos at risk of developmental arrest or improper zona thinning[6]

Contd...

Contd...

Parameter	*Description*	*Impact on ART outcomes*	*Solution*
Inner cell mass morphology	The ICM should ideally be compact, cohesive, and centrally localized within the blastocyst cavity. Its position and structural integrity are indicative of proper embryonic differentiation and viability. When the ICM appears dispersed, loosely packed, localized peripherally rather than centrally, or shows signs of degeneration, it suggests compromised pluripotent potential, suboptimal culture conditions, or increased cellular apoptosis—all of which may negatively impact implantation and developmental outcomes	High-quality ICM is linked to better embryo viability, higher implantation rates, and greater differentiation potential. Poor ICM morphology is often linked to mitochondrial dysfunction or chromosomal imbalances affecting early cell differentiation	Implement noninvasive imaging techniques like optical coherence tomography (OCT) or fluorescence-based markers for mitochondrial health assessment to evaluate ICM quality. Optimize embryo culture conditions, including the use of low-oxygen (5%) culture environments and antioxidant supplementation, to support ICM formation and minimize stress-induced damage
Trophectoderm quality	The TE layer should consist of a uniform layer of cohesive cells lining the outer blastocyst surface. Poor-quality TE appears fragmented, uneven, or vacuolated, often indicating suboptimal cellular function or compromised cytoskeletal integrity	TE quality is directly correlated with implantation potential, as it forms the placenta and interfaces with the maternal endometrium. Poor TE morphology leads to lower implantation rates, impaired placental development, and increased miscarriage risk	Optimize culture conditions, including proper glucose and amino acid concentrations, to support TE integrity. Consider noninvasive metabolomic profiling to assess cellular health and predict TE quality[6]
Blastocyst grading (Gardner's criteria)	Grading includes assessment of blastocyst expansion (graded 1–6), ICM quality (graded A–C), and TE quality (graded A–C). High-grade blastocysts (AA or AB) show full expansion and have cohesive, well-defined ICM and TE layers	High-grade blastocysts are associated with higher implantation rates and live birth outcomes, while low-grade blastocysts (e.g., grade C ICM or TE) have reduced developmental potential and increased risk of implantation failure or developmental arrest	Use strict grading criteria based on Gardner's system to ensure accurate assessment and selection of high-quality embryos. Regularly calibrate grading among embryologists to ensure consistency and reliability in evaluating blastocyst quality. Implement quality assurance programs to maintain high interlaboratory grading accuracy[6]

(ART: assisted reproductive technology)

TABLE 3: Common morphological and developmental abnormalities during embryo assessment and their impact on ART outcomes.

Issue	*Description*	*Impact on ART outcomes*	*Solution*
Localized and percentage fragmentation	Fragmentation results from apoptotic processes, compromised cell-cycle regulation, or oxidative stress. Localized fragments (e.g., central or peripheral) and high fragmentation percentage (>25%) are detrimental and suggest compromised embryo health	High fragmentation is associated with reduced cell communication, impaired metabolic function, and increased risk of aneuploidy or implantation failure	Use antiapoptotic agents (e.g., caspase inhibitors) or low-oxygen culture conditions to reduce fragmentation. Monitor fragmentation dynamics using time-lapse imaging to identify transient versus permanent fragmentation. Implement early transfer or vitrification of embryos with moderate fragmentation levels (<25%) if they show good cleavage patterns and minimal cytoplasmic abnormalities[4]
Blastomere degeneration	Blastomere degeneration may be due to mitochondrial dysfunction, failed DNA repair, or exposure to environmental stressors like temperature fluctuations or light exposure	Degeneration reduces blastocyst formation rates and compromises cellular communication. It often indicates genetic abnormalities or impaired energy production	Use antioxidants like CoQ10 or resveratrol to enhance mitochondrial function and counteract oxidative damage. Implement quality control measures to maintain stable environmental conditions during embryo culture. Consider noninvasive metabolic profiling to assess energy production and identify embryos at risk of degeneration[3]
Asymmetrical blastomere division	Unequal division of blastomeres is a sign of chromosomal imbalances, spindle defects, or cytoskeletal disorganization. It disrupts the balance of blastomere sizes, leading to developmental arrest or abnormal blastocyst formation	Asymmetrical division patterns can affect blastocyst quality and are associated with higher rates of implantation failure and genetic abnormalities, such as mosaicism or trisomy	Use genetic testing techniques like preimplantation genetic testing for aneuploidy (PGT-A) to identify chromosomal imbalances. Monitor cell division using time-lapse technology to detect irregularities and decide on the best transfer time or vitrification strategy. Implement spindle checkpoint analysis to evaluate cell-cycle progression[1]
Sudden developmental arrest	Sudden developmental arrest occurs when an embryo abruptly stops dividing due to factors like chromosomal abnormalities, metabolic failure, or oxidative stress. It can occur at any stage but is most observed at the 8-cell stage or during early blastocyst formation	Developmental arrest is a sign of severe chromosomal abnormalities or metabolic dysfunction and indicates no further developmental potential. Arrested embryos are nonviable and unsuitable for transfer or cryopreservation	Implement genetic screening techniques, such as PGT-A or whole-genome sequencing (WGS), to identify genetic causes of arrest. Use noninvasive biomarkers, such as mitochondrial activity or ROS levels, to monitor metabolic health. Optimize culture conditions, including oxygen concentration (5%) and temperature, to minimize stress[6]

Contd...

Contd...

Issue	*Description*	*Impact on ART outcomes*	*Solution*
Cytoplasmic abnormalities	Cytoplasmic abnormalities, such as vacuoles, granules, or dark inclusions, indicate cytoplasmic stress, poor organelle distribution, or metabolic imbalances. They are often linked to mitochondrial dysfunction or abnormal protein synthesis[5]	Cytoplasmic abnormalities are associated with poor blastocyst quality, increased rates of developmental arrest, and reduced implantation potential	Implement metabolic profiling to detect abnormalities in protein synthesis and mitochondrial activity. Use optimized media formulations to support cellular health and minimize environmental stress during culture[3]

(ART: assisted reproductive technology; ROS: reactive oxygen species)

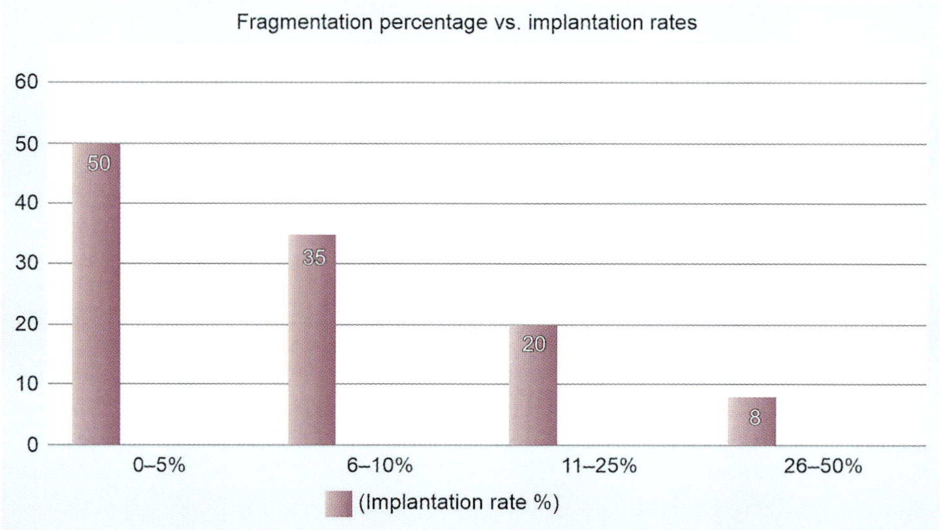

Fig. 1: Impact of embryo fragmentation on implantation success rates.

(Table 4). Disruptions in these processes can lead to developmental arrest, poor-quality embryos, or implantation failure.

EMBRYO SELECTION

Embryo selection is a carefully individualized process guided by a combination of embryological observations and patient-specific clinical parameters. While morphological grading based on blastomere symmetry, fragmentation, developmental stage, and cytoplasmic characteristics remains central, decisions must also factor in maternal age, previous cycle history, ovarian response, and the readiness and receptivity of the endometrium. Embryos should be selected at the most appropriate developmental stage; neither too delayed nor excessively advanced, since abnormal timing can reflect compromised developmental potential. In some countries, laws may regulate the number or type of embryos that can be transferred or cultured to later stages. Additionally, time-lapse imaging,

TABLE 4: Molecular and biochemical determinants of embryo arrest and blastocyst development in ART.

Factor	*Description*	*Impact on ART outcomes*	*Solution*
Genetic mutations and translation errors	Mutations in genes regulating cell division, cytoskeletal dynamics, and energy metabolism can disrupt protein synthesis and translation, leading to impaired embryo development. Mutations in genes like *PLK4, AURKB,* or *POU5F1* can severely compromise cleavage and blastocyst formation	Genetic mutations cause developmental arrest, asymmetric division, or chromosomal anomalies, lowering implantation potential and increasing the risk of implantation failure or early miscarriage	Use genetic testing techniques like whole-genome sequencing (WGS) or targeted sequencing to identify mutations affecting embryo development. Implement oocyte and sperm selection based on genetic screening results. Optimize culture conditions and media to minimize stress-induced mutations during embryonic development[7]
Stage-specific protein synthesis	Protein synthesis and expression vary at different stages of embryo development, with critical proteins required for processes such as cleavage, compaction, and blastocyst formation. Disruptions in stage-specific protein synthesis can impede cell division and differentiation, leading to developmental arrest. Errors in the expression of key proteins like E-cadherin, ZO-1, or OCT-4 can severely affect embryo morphology and function	Errors in protein synthesis or translation are linked to abnormal cleavage patterns, poor blastocyst formation, and failed differentiation. Embryos with impaired protein synthesis often show signs of developmental arrest or poor-quality ICM and TE formation.	Monitor protein synthesis using noninvasive proteomic analysis or transcriptomic profiling to assess stage-specific expression patterns. Use media supplemented with growth factors like IGF-1 or FGF-2 to support protein synthesis and cellular communication during critical stages of development. Use time-lapse imaging to correlate protein synthesis patterns with morphokinetic events[8]
Oxidative stress and redox potential	Elevated oxidative stress leads to DNA damage, impaired cellular signaling, and reduced energy production, compromising embryo viability. High redox potential can disrupt spindle formation, induce DNA fragmentation, and impair mitochondrial function. Elevated ROS levels are often observed in embryos with poor developmental potential.	High oxidative stress and poor redox regulation are linked to increased DNA fragmentation, lower implantation rates, and reduced embryo quality. Embryos exposed to high oxidative stress have higher rates of developmental arrest and reduced blastocyst formation.	Use antioxidants like melatonin, CoQ10, or resveratrol in culture systems to reduce oxidative stress. Implement noninvasive metabolic assays to assess mitochondrial function and oxidative damage. Optimize environmental conditions (e.g., oxygen concentration, temperature, and light exposure) to minimize oxidative stress during embryo culture.[4]

Contd...

Contd...

Factor	*Description*	*Impact on ART outcomes*	*Solution*
Cytoskeletal dynamics and morphokinetics	Cytoskeletal organization is crucial for cell division, blastomere symmetry, and blastocyst expansion. Disruption in cytoskeletal dynamics can result in irregular cleavage patterns, fragmentation, or developmental arrest. Mutations or disruptions in cytoskeletal proteins like actin, tubulin, or myosin impair cellular organization and division	Abnormal cytoskeletal organization can cause cleavage arrest, asymmetric division, and poor blastocyst quality. Embryos with compromised cytoskeletal integrity often show signs of fragmentation, vacuolation, or irregular blastomere sizes, reducing implantation potential and viability	Implement protocols to stabilize cytoskeletal dynamics, such as maintaining optimal osmolarity and calcium regulation in culture media. Use cytoskeletal-stabilizing agents like taxol or cytochalasin B at appropriate concentrations to support cytoskeletal health during critical stages of development[3]

(ART: assisted reproductive technology; FGF-2: fibroblast growth factor 2; ICM: inner cell mass; IGF-1: insulin-like growth factor 1; ROS: reactive oxygen species)

metabolic profiling, and genetic testing may aid in refining selection when available. Thus, embryo selection is not based on appearance alone but represents a multidisciplinary judgment aimed at choosing the embryo with the best chance for successful implantation and healthy pregnancy.

CONCLUSION

Embryo assessment is a multifaceted process that plays a pivotal role in determining the success of ART procedures. By meticulously evaluating morphological parameters—such as blastomere symmetry, fragmentation, and blastocyst expansion—as well as biochemical and genetic markers, embryologists gain critical insights into the developmental potential and viability of embryos. Understanding the complexities of embryo development at different stages, from Day 3 cleavage to Day 5 blastocyst formation, allows for the identification of high-quality embryos with optimal implantation potential. Moreover, addressing common issues like asynchronous cleavage, degeneration, cytoplasmic abnormalities, or developmental arrest through targeted troubleshooting strategies can significantly improve outcomes. Incorporating advanced diagnostic tools, such as time-lapse imaging and genetic screening, alongside a deep understanding of cellular biochemistry, enables more precise embryo selection and personalized treatment plans. Ultimately, an integrated approach to embryo assessment—combining morphology, biochemistry, and genetics—not only enhances the efficiency of ART but also improves clinical success rates, bringing patients closer to achieving their goal of a successful pregnancy and healthy birth.

REFERENCES

1. Van den Berg M, Overwater C. Impact of blastomere asymmetry on embryo development and live birth rates in IVF/ICSI cycles. Reprod BioMed Online. 2019;39(3):437-46.
2. Alpha Scientists in Reproductive Medicine. The Istanbul consensus workshop on embryo

assessment: Proceedings of an expert meeting. Reprod BioMed Online. 2011;22(6): 632-46.
3. Rienzi L, Ubaldi FM, Iacobelli M. Optimizing human oocyte cryopreservation: An analysis of the current state of the art. J Clin Endocrinol Metabol. 2019;104(4):1469-79.
4. Balaban B, Brison D, Calderon G. The development of morphological assessment criteria for human embryo development and their value in predicting pregnancy and live birth outcomes. Hum Reprod Update. 2011;17(5):485-503.
5. Abbott AL, Fissore RA, Ducibella T. The role of cortical granules in fertilization and polyspermy prevention. J Reprod Immunol. 2015;108:1-7.
6. Gardner DK, Schoolcraft WB. In vitro culture of human blastocysts. Clin Obstet Gynecol. 2013;43(4):705-21.
7. De Rycke M, Bergh C, Mertes H. Biopsy-related risks for human embryo and fetus: Time to change the focus. Hum Reprod Update. 2020;26(4):470-92.
8. Wai T, Ao A, Zhang X, Pinto M. The role of mitochondrial mutations in male infertility. Hum Reprod Update. 2010;16(2):143-58.

SECTION

4 Culture, Cryopreservation, and Transfer

CHAPTER

11

Culture Systems

INTRODUCTION

In assisted reproductive technology (ART), culture systems are the cornerstone of success, as they provide the essential environment for gamete maturation, fertilization, and embryo development. These systems must be finely tuned to regulate factors such as temperature, pH, CO_2 levels, humidity, and media composition. Even minor deviations in these parameters can disrupt cellular processes, leading to problems such as slow cleavage, developmental arrest, increased fragmentation, or apoptosis. Moreover, maintaining sterility and preventing contamination are crucial to ensuring the quality and viability of embryos. This chapter covers the key components of ART culture systems, including media selection, environmental control, sterility management, and the use of specific substances such as oil overlays, hyaluronidase, and polyvinylpyrrolidone (PVP), along with troubleshooting strategies based on the latest scientific insights.

MEDIA TYPES AND COMPOSITION IN ASSISTED REPRODUCTIVE TECHNOLOGY CULTURE SYSTEMS

Culture media serve as the foundation of any ART culture system, providing the necessary nutrients, energy sources, and biochemical support for embryos as they transition from fertilization to blastocyst formation **(Table 1)**. The two most common types of media used in ART are sequential and one-step media, each designed to address different metabolic needs during various stages of development **(Table 2)**.

AMINO ACIDS, ETHYLENEDIAMINETETRAACETIC ACID, AND ANTIBIOTICS IN CULTURE MEDIA

- *Amino acids (AAs):* Amino acids serve as key metabolic substrates and regulators of embryo development. In early cleavage

TABLE 1: Amino acids (AAs) types in culture media and their functions.

Amino acid type	*Examples*	*Function in embryo culture*
Nonessential AAs	Alanine, glutamine, and glycine	Early cleavage support, osmotic regulation, and energy source
Essential AAs	Leucine, lysine, and methionine	Required for blastocyst development and protein synthesis
Glutamine	Glutamine and glutamate	Cell proliferation and antioxidant protection
Taurine and hypotaurine	Modified AA derivatives	ROS scavenging and membrane stability
EDTA	Chelating agent	Reduces ROS, and protects early embryos

(EDTA: ethylenediaminetetraacetic acid; ROS: reactive oxygen species)

TABLE 2: Sequential versus one-step media.

Media type	*Description*	*Impact on ART outcomes*	*Solution*
Sequential media	Sequential media are designed to match the changing metabolic needs of embryos as they progress through different stages. One medium supports early cleavage stages, while another is used during the blastocyst stage	Sequential media provide optimal conditions for each developmental stage, mimicking the in vivo environment. However, the need for dish changes introduces risks such as handling errors, exposure to air, and contamination[1]	Minimize embryo handling by streamlining dish changes and reducing exposure time. Pre-equilibrate media thoroughly and maintain stable environmental conditions, including CO_2 and temperature, to avoid stress on the embryos during transitions[2]
One-step media	One-step media maintain embryos in a single culture medium from fertilization through to the blastocyst stage, containing nutrients, amino acids, and growth factors that support development throughout	One-step media reduce the need for handling, lowering the risk of contamination and embryo stress. However, pH and nutrient stability may become challenging during extended culture periods[3]	Use one-step media when minimal handling is required, such as in time-lapse incubators. Ensure that the media are fully equilibrated before use to maintain stable pH levels. Implement oil overlays to protect against evaporation and pH fluctuations[4]

stages, nonessential amino acids such as glycine, taurine, and alanine help to regulate osmolarity, support protein synthesis, and reduce ammonia accumulation. In contrast, essential amino acids such as glutamine, leucine, and isoleucine become more critical during the morula to blastocyst transition, where cellular proliferation and differentiation intensify. Amino acids also act as carbon and nitrogen sources, influencing energy metabolism and nucleic acid synthesis.[1]

- *Ethylenediaminetetraacetic acid (EDTA):* EDTA functions as a metal ion chelator, binding divalent cations like Fe^{2+} and Cu^{2+} to prevent the formation of reactive oxygen species (ROS). This protects preimplantation embryos from oxidative stress, especially during early cleavage stages when endogenous antioxidant systems are immature. EDTA also serves as a free radical scavenger, maintaining redox balance and aiding in the preservation of genomic integrity.[3]
- *Antibiotics:* Antibiotics such as gentamicin and streptomycin are included to prevent bacterial contamination, especially during long-term culture. However, their presence must be tightly regulated, as high concentrations may interfere with mitochondrial translation, protein synthesis, and cellular respiration. Overuse can inadvertently suppress beneficial microbiota or compromise embryo metabolism. Therefore, batch validation and sterility assurance of media is crucial to limit antibiotic reliance while maintaining contamination-free environments.[5]
- *Buffers and pH regulators:* Most culture media use a bicarbonate buffer system in conjunction with controlled CO_2 atmospheres to maintain physiological pH (7.2–7.4). 4-(2-hydroxyethyl)-1-piperazineethanesulfonic acid (HEPES) or 3-(N-morpholino) propanesulfonic acid (MOPS) buffers are also employed in handling media outside CO_2 incubators, offering pH stability during procedures like

intracytoplasmic sperm injection (ICSI) or embryo transfer.

- *Hormones and growth factors:* Although not always included in standard IVF media, some advanced media formulations contain epidermal growth factor (EGF), insulin, or recombinant gonadotropins to mimic in vivo signaling pathways. These factors may enhance metabolic activation, compaction, and blastocyst formation when supplemented appropriately.
- *Scavengers and antioxidants:* In addition to EDTA, media may be supplemented with glutathione, vitamin C, vitamin E, or melatonin, which serve as ROS scavengers to reduce oxidative injury during in vitro development. These agents help to stabilize mitochondrial function, protect lipids and DNA, and promote healthier embryonic development under in vitro conditions.

ENVIRONMENTAL CONTROL IN CULTURE SYSTEMS

Maintaining precise environmental conditions is essential for optimal oocyte and embryo development. Critical parameters such as pH (ideally 7.2–7.4), CO_2 concentration (5–6% for bicarbonate-buffered media), humidity (≥95%), and temperature (37°C) must be tightly regulated to prevent cellular stress and developmental arrest. Oocytes, particularly during the metaphase II stage, are highly sensitive to temperature fluctuations and pH shifts, which can compromise spindle integrity and cytoplasmic maturation. During the precompaction stage (Days 1–3), embryos rely on low oxygen conditions (5% O_2) and benefit from media supplemented with nonessential amino acids and EDTA to support cleavage without premature differentiation. In contrast, postcompaction embryos (Days 4–6) exhibit increased metabolic demands and require essential amino acids, antioxidants, and higher glucose concentrations to support blastocyst expansion and lineage specification. Ensuring a stable and embryo-safe environment throughout these transitions is crucial for maintaining viability, minimizing ROS, and supporting successful implantation.

CO_2 LEVELS AND pH STABILITY

CO_2 plays a vital role in maintaining the pH balance of bicarbonate-buffered culture media. Fluctuations in CO_2 levels can lead to pH instability, which adversely affects metabolic functions, protein synthesis, and cell division **(Table 3)**.

HUMIDITY AND TEMPERATURE CONTROL

Humidity and temperature must remain stable to prevent cellular stress and media evaporation. Any fluctuations in temperature can result in thermal shock, which can damage the meiotic spindle of oocytes and disrupt mitotic divisions in embryos. Similarly, low humidity can cause evaporation of culture media, leading to changes in osmolarity and pH, ultimately compromising embryo viability. External factors such as altitude and geographical location can influence ambient pressure and humidity levels, necessitating site-specific adjustments in incubator calibration and room design. The use of dehumidifiers, air conditioning systems, or room heaters must be carefully balanced, as they can inadvertently reduce room humidity or cause temperature fluctuations if not properly maintained or calibrated. Therefore, maintaining a controlled laboratory environment with continuous monitoring, sealed equipment, minimal air turbulence, and appropriate insulation is essential to preserve the stability of embryo culture conditions and ensure optimal outcomes **(Table 4)**.

TABLE 3: Gas and pH control parameters in embryo culture systems.

Parameter	*Description*	*Impact on ART outcomes*	*Solution*
CO_2 concentration	CO_2 levels typically range from 5 to 6% in ART culture systems, regulating pH in bicarbonate-buffered media. Incubator malfunctions or inconsistencies in gas supply can cause CO_2 fluctuations	CO_2 variations lead to pH imbalances, affecting enzyme activity, mitochondrial function, and nutrient transport. This can result in slow cleavage, increased fragmentation, and developmental arrest[2]	Regularly calibrate CO_2 incubators to ensure proper functioning. Use external sensors to monitor CO_2 levels continuously. Use sealed culture dishes with oil overlays to protect against pH fluctuations caused by air exposure[3]
pH variation	pH is sensitive to environmental changes, and small variations in CO_2 levels or prolonged exposure to air can disrupt pH balance in culture media. The optimal pH for embryo culture is 7.2–7.4	pH fluctuations increase oxidative stress, disrupt mitochondrial activity, and impair nutrient uptake, leading to poor blastocyst formation and increased apoptosis[5]	Use oil overlays to stabilize pH and minimize exposure to ambient air. Monitor pH regularly using microelectrodes or dyes to detect deviations early. Pre-equilibrate media in incubators to maintain stable pH levels[4]

TABLE 4: Humidity and temperature regulation in embryo culture systems.

Parameter	*Description*	*Impact on ART outcomes*	*Solution*
Humidity control	Maintaining humidity at 95% helps to prevent evaporation of culture media, which maintains stable osmolarity and nutrient concentrations	Low humidity leads to evaporation, which alters media composition and osmotic balance, causing osmotic stress to embryos and increasing the risk of fragmentation[2]	Ensure that incubators have humidity control systems. Use oil overlays to protect media from evaporation. Regularly check the osmolarity of culture media to ensure it remains consistent, adjusting humidity settings as necessary[5]
Temperature control	Embryos require a constant temperature of 37°C for optimal cellular function. Deviations can disrupt metabolic and genetic processes	Temperature fluctuations result in cellular damage, reduced cleavage rates, and an increase in apoptosis. Improper temperature control can lead to failed embryo development[6]	Use temperature-controlled workstations and prewarmed media to avoid thermal shock. Regularly calibrate incubators and heating blocks to maintain consistent temperature. Monitor temperature with real-time sensors to detect and correct deviations promptly[1]

STERILITY AND CONTAMINATION CONTROL IN ASSISTED REPRODUCTIVE TECHNOLOGY CULTURE SYSTEMS

Ensuring sterility in ART culture systems is fundamental to preserving embryo viability, as any form of contamination whether microbial, particulate like cotton fibers, or chemical such as endotoxins can severely disrupt the delicate in vitro environment. The quality of consumables plays a pivotal role, and only medical-grade, embryo-tested plastics with appropriate transparency or minimal opacity should be used to ensure both sterility and visual clarity during micromanipulation. Improperly manufactured or stored consumables can leach toxic substances or harbor residual contaminants, posing a serious threat to gamete and embryo health. Sterility must be validated not just by manufacturer certifications such as gamma irradiation, but also through in-laboratory disinfection practices and using sterile packaging within designated clean zones. Additionally, culture media and consumables must be lot-tested prior to use, since variations even between batches can affect embryo development. Decontamination workflows should include the use of incubators with HEPA filters, aseptic workstation design, validated entry protocols, and scheduled sterility monitoring. Maintaining sterility is thus a dynamic and proactive process, requiring continuous vigilance, standardized protocols, and consistent quality checks across all stages of the IVF workflow **(Table 5)**.

OILS, HYALURONIDASE, AND POLYVINYLPYRROLIDONE IN ASSISTED REPRODUCTIVE TECHNOLOGY CULTURE SYSTEMS

In addition to media, specific substances like oil overlays **(Table 6)**, hyaluronidase (hylase) **(Table 7)**, and PVP **(Table 8)** play crucial roles in protecting media, facilitating sperm selection, and aiding in oocyte denudation during ART procedures **(Table 9)**.

MONITORING EMBRYO DEVELOPMENT: CLEAVAGE, FRAGMENTATION, AND APOPTOSIS

Embryo development must be closely monitored throughout the culture period to assess the health of the embryos and identify potential issues such as abnormal cleavage, fragmentation, and apoptosis **(Table 10)**. These indicators are critical for selecting high-quality embryos for transfer.

TABLE 5: Contamination from particulates and inadequate sterilization in assisted reproductive technology (ART) laboratories.

Source of contamination	*Description*	*Impact on ART outcomes*	*Solution*
Cotton fibers and particulates	Cotton fibers, dust, and other particulates can enter culture dishes during handling, introducing contaminants that interfere with media composition and embryo development	Physical contaminants can damage embryos, disrupt sperm-oocyte interactions, and introduce microbial organisms that affect fertilization and embryo quality[7]	Use lint-free materials in the laboratory, and avoid cotton-based laboratory coats and towels. Implement strict gowning protocols, and inspect culture dishes for visible contaminants before use. Use filtered pipette tips and sterile workstations to prevent contamination[6]
Disinfection and sterilization protocols	Inadequate sterilization of media, dishes, and tools introduces microbial contaminants that compromise embryo health. Even trace amounts of endotoxins can impair embryo development	Contaminated media lead to increased apoptosis, poor-quality embryos, and failed implantation. Endotoxins disrupt normal cellular processes, leading to developmental arrest[7]	Use sterile, single-use culture dishes and autoclave reusable tools. Conduct regular microbiological testing, such as endotoxin assays, to validate the sterility of culture media and tools. Employ UV sterilization of incubators and workstations to maintain contamination-free environments[5]

TABLE 6: Comparative assessment of oil types used in ART culture systems.

Oil type	*Description*	*Impact on ART outcomes*	*Solution*
Liquid paraffin	Liquid paraffin is commonly used to overlay culture media to protect against evaporation and maintain stable temperature and pH	Liquid paraffin effectively stabilizes the culture environment, but poorly purified oil can introduce toxic compounds that harm embryos, such as peroxides and VOCs[1]	Use highly purified, sterile-filtered liquid paraffin and pre-equilibrate the oil in incubators before use. Regularly test oil for toxicity using mouse embryo assays (MEA) to ensure it supports normal embryo development[2]
Mineral oil	Mineral oil is another commonly used overlay with a higher viscosity, offering better protection for smaller culture droplets	Mineral oil maintains pH and temperature stability, but its higher viscosity can complicate handling during ICSI. Contaminated oil introduces risks of microbial contamination and VOC exposure[4]	Prewarm mineral oil and ensure it is fully sterile before use. Choose an oil with appropriate viscosity based on the size of the culture droplet and the procedure **(Fig. 1)**, such as ICSI or embryo culture[2]

(ART: assisted reproductive technology; ICSI: intracytoplasmic sperm injection; VOCs: volatile organic compounds)

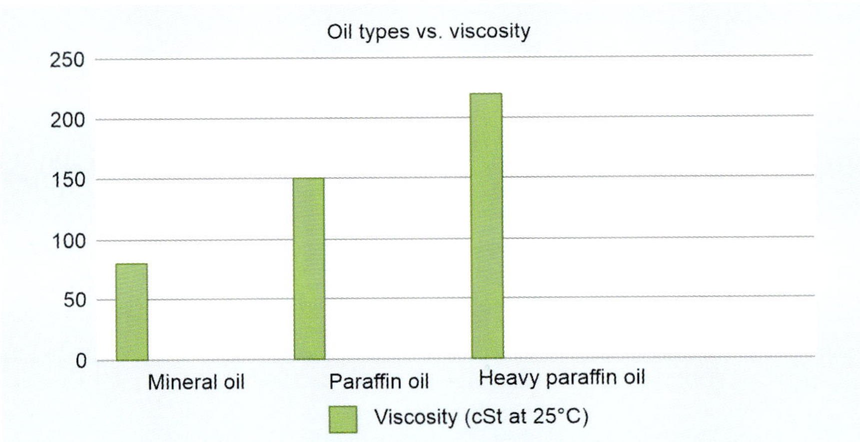

Fig. 1: Comparative viscosity of different oil types used in embryo culture systems.

TABLE 7: Hyaluronidase (Hylase) in oocyte denudation.

Substance	*Description*	*Impact on ART outcomes*	*Solution*
Hyaluronidase (Hylase)	Hyaluronidase is used to break down the extracellular matrix in cumulus cells surrounding oocytes, facilitating denudation prior to ICSI	Proper use of hyaluronidase aids in gentle and efficient removal of cumulus cells. Overexposure, however, can damage the oocyte's zona pellucida and cytoplasm, compromising fertilization rates[8]	Limit exposure time to hyaluronidase (1–2 minutes at 80 IU/mL is typical) and rinse oocytes thoroughly in fresh media after denudation. Minimize mechanical stress on oocytes during denudation to preserve cell viability[4]

(ART: assisted reproductive technology; ICSI: intracytoplasmic sperm injection)

TABLE 8: Polyvinylpyrrolidone (PVP) in ICSI.

Substance	*Description*	*Impact on ART outcomes*	*Solution*
Polyvinylpyrrolidone	PVP is a viscous polymer solution used to immobilize sperm during ICSI, making sperm easier to select and inject. Concentrations of 7 and 10% PVP are commonly used depending on the viscosity required, with 10% offering more stable immobilization for precise handling. However, care must be taken during injection to avoid introducing excess PVP into the oocyte, as deposition of the polymer can affect ooplasmic integrity and disrupt fertilization	PVP facilitates sperm immobilization, but prolonged exposure can damage sperm DNA and reduce viability. Overexposure also increases the risk of sperm sticking to the pipette, complicating the injection process[6]	Use PVP with caution, limiting sperm exposure to only a few minutes before injection. Always ensure that PVP is prepared and tested for purity to avoid introducing contaminants during ICSI. Proper handling techniques should be used to minimize damage to the sperm[8]

(ART: assisted reproductive technology; ICSI: intracytoplasmic sperm injection)

TABLE 9: Oil types—viscosity, overlay behavior, and batch variability.

Oil type	*Viscosity (cSt at 25°C)*	*Overlay behavior*	*Batch variability*	*Notes*
Mineral oil	65–100	Lighter, less dense, and faster spread	High (natural source)	Risk of peroxides; less commonly used today
Paraffin oil	120–200	Heavier and stable overlay	Low (synthetic source)	Preferred in IVF; undergoes filtration and QC
Heavy paraffin oil	>200	Slow spread, and minimal evaporation loss	Low	Used for long-term culture

(IVF: in-vitro fertilization; QC: quality control)

CONCLUSION

Culture systems in ART are essential for creating an optimal environment that supports gamete maturation, fertilization, and embryo development. Maintaining precise control over factors such as media composition, pH, CO_2 levels, temperature, and sterility is critical to ensuring successful outcomes. The selection of appropriate media, whether sequential or one-step, and the careful use of substances like hyaluronidase and PVP during procedures like ICSI, play a crucial role in minimizing stress on gametes and embryos. Environmental stability, including humidity and temperature control, is vital for preventing issues such as developmental arrest, fragmentation, or apoptosis. Troubleshooting culture systems involve constant monitoring and swift intervention to correct deviations, ultimately improving fertilization rates, embryo quality, and clinical success.

TABLE 10: Embryo developmental kinetics and quality markers in assisted reproductive technology (ART).

Parameter	*Description*	*Impact on ART outcomes*	*Solution*
Cleavage rate	The cleavage rate refers to the timing of cell division in the developing embryo. Normal cleavage follows a consistent timeline (e.g., 2-cell at 24 hours, 8-cell at 72 hours)	Abnormally slow or fast cleavage can indicate metabolic stress, suboptimal culture conditions, or genetic abnormalities, which are associated with lower implantation rates and increased risk of miscarriage[2]	Monitor cleavage rates using time-lapse imaging to track real-time development and detect deviations early. Adjust culture media composition to provide necessary metabolic support. Ensure stable pH and temperature conditions throughout the culture period[4]
Fragmentation	Fragmentation involves the separation of small cytoplasmic pieces within the embryo. Low fragmentation (below 15%) is common, but higher levels (>25%) suggest significant developmental stress	High fragmentation is linked to chromosomal anomalies, poor embryo quality, and lower implantation rates. It may result from oxidative stress, improper media composition, or suboptimal environmental conditions[7]	Regularly monitor fragmentation levels and assess the cause of stress. Use antioxidant-supplemented media to reduce oxidative stress. Optimize culture conditions, including pH and temperature, and reduce handling times to minimize stress on developing embryos[1]
Apoptosis	Apoptosis is the process of programmed cell death. While it occurs naturally in developing embryos, excessive apoptosis is indicative of cellular damage or stress	High levels of apoptosis lead to poor-quality embryos, developmental arrest, and reduced implantation rates. Apoptosis may be triggered by oxidative stress, genetic mutations, or disruptions in culture conditions[6]	Use culture media with antioxidants, such as melatonin or vitamin C, to protect embryos from oxidative stress. Monitor environmental factors such as temperature, pH, and CO_2 levels to ensure stability. Genetic screening of embryos may help to identify underlying mutations that contribute to apoptosis[4]
Time-lapse monitoring	Time-lapse imaging tracks embryo development in real-time, allowing for detailed observation of cleavage, fragmentation, and abnormal cellular events without disturbing the culture environment	Time-lapse monitoring provides early detection of abnormal development patterns, allowing for better embryo selection. This leads to improved implantation rates and reduced miscarriage risk[4]	Implement time-lapse monitoring systems in the laboratory to continuously assess embryo development. Use the detailed data provided by these systems to guide embryo selection and optimize culture conditions[1]

REFERENCES

1. Gardner DK, Lane M. Embryo culture systems: Role of media, gas environment, and temperature. Fertil Steril. 2013;99(4):856-62.
2. Gardner DK, Kelley RL. Embryo culture systems: Optimization for ART outcomes. Reprod BioMed Online. 2018;36(4):387-96.
3. Biggers JD, Summers MC. Choosing a culture medium: Making informed decisions. Fertil Steril. 2008;90(2):473-83.
4. Esfandiari N, Nazemian Z. Impact of culture systems on in vitro fertilization outcomes. J Assist Reprod Genetics. 2017;34(10):1345-54.
5. Menezo Y, Dale B. Embryo environment and quality: The importance of the microenvironment. Reprod BioMed Online. 2013;27(5):402-11.
6. Van den Bergh M, Overwater C. Influence of PVP on sperm DNA integrity during ICSI. Reprod Biomed Online. 2016;32(4):398-404.
7. Vermesh M, Samo M, Saadat P. Reducing contamination in ART: Air quality and microbiological monitoring. Fertil Steril. 2020;113(3):519-29.
8. Swain JE, Lai D, Takayama S, Smith GD. Thinking big by thinking small: Application of microfluidic technology to improve ART. Lab on a Chip. 2012;12(7):1214-20.

CHAPTER

12

Cryopreservation

INTRODUCTION

Cryopreservation is a cornerstone of assisted reproductive technology (ART), enabling flexible cycle scheduling, fertility preservation, and improved cumulative pregnancy rates without repeated ovarian stimulation. Both slow freezing and vitrification techniques are utilized depending on cell type, with vitrification now being the preferred method for oocytes and embryos due to its superior survival and developmental outcomes. Oocyte vitrification requires careful equilibration in basal solutions supplemented with appropriate cryoprotectant agents (CPA) [e.g., ethylene glycol (EG), dimethyl sulfoxide (DMSO), and sucrose], due to their sensitivity to osmotic shifts and their lack of protective cumulus cells. Embryos, particularly blastocysts, are more robust but still vulnerable to ice crystal formation if cooling and warming rates are not optimal. While the efficiency of vitrification and warming has advanced, the process remains vulnerable to subtle variations in cellular physiology, cryoprotectant interactions, and laboratory environmental control.[1] Suboptimal cryopreservation can lead to reduced post-thaw viability, spindle damage in oocytes, zona hardening, mitochondrial dysfunction, and developmental arrest.[2] Maintaining consistent loading techniques, temperature regulation, and timing across cryopreservation steps is critical for preserving cellular integrity and maximizing clinical success.

CELLULAR RESPONSE TO CRYOPRESERVATION

The freezing and thawing process imposes extreme stress on cells. Effective preservation depends on limiting intracellular ice formation, controlling osmotic shock, and avoiding cryoprotectant toxicity **(Table 1)**. Parameters

TABLE 1: Cellular determinants influencing cryopreservation efficacy.

Factor	*Scientific impact on cells*	*Recommendations*
Cell volume	Larger cells like oocytes have a lower surface-to-volume ratio, increasing the risk of intracellular ice formation[4]	Use higher concentrations of permeable cryoprotectants like DMSO or EG, with optimized equilibration time[5]
Surface area	Greater surface area enhances membrane permeability, aiding CPA diffusion[3]	Denude oocytes completely before vitrification to promote uniform CPA entry
Membrane permeability	Membrane lipid composition influences the rate of CPA and water exchange[3]	Calibrate protocols for specific cell types (e.g., oocytes and blastocysts); avoid abrupt dehydration[5]
Cytoskeletal sensitivity	Microtubules and meiotic spindles are temperature-sensitive and depolymerize rapidly at low temperatures[6]	Maintain stable temperatures during handling; avoid prolonged exposure to 4–15°C

(CPA: cryoprotectant agent; DMSO: dimethyl sulfoxide; EG: ethylene glycol)

such as cell volume, membrane properties, and cytoskeletal resilience influence how cells tolerate cryopreservation.[3]

CRYOPROTECTANTS: COMPOSITION, TOXICITY, AND TIMING

Cryoprotectants work by displacing intracellular water and increasing viscosity, which prevents ice crystal formation and promotes vitrification. Common agents like EG, DMSO, and propanediol protect cells during freezing, but their cytotoxicity increases with prolonged exposure or incorrect combinations.[2] These solutions are typically packaged in sterile plastic or glass vials, either translucent or opaque, with variations in density and light protection depending on the manufacturer. Their storage and handling conditions are critical, as repeated temperature fluctuations can degrade their efficacy. Though essential for oocyte and embryo cryopreservation, especially in vitrification, careful adherence to exposure timing is necessary to avoid cellular damage, including mitochondrial injury, zona hardening, or spindle disruption **(Table 2)**.[5]

VITRIFICATION AND WARMING PROTOCOLS: TIMING AND EXPOSURE

Protocol precision is vital to successful cryopreservation **(Table 3)**. Vitrification avoids crystallization by ultrarapid cooling, but errors during equilibration, solution transition, or warming can be catastrophic.[9]

TABLE 2: Cryoprotectant agents (CPAs): Function, limitations, and optimization strategies.

CPA	*Function*	*Common issues*	*Solution*
Dimethyl sulfoxide (DMSO)	Rapid membrane penetration with moderate toxicity	May cause DNA fragmentation and epigenetic changes	Keep exposure below 1 minute; use fresh, prewarmed solutions and validate for toxicity
Ethylene glycol (EG)	Lower toxicity and slower permeability	Osmotic imbalance and delayed permeation	Combine with DMSO; pre-equilibrate; maintain temperature consistency[7]
Sucrose	Osmotic buffer aiding dehydration	Incomplete dehydration → intracellular ice	Use stepwise concentrations; follow with isotonic washing postwarming[6]
Propanediol	Slow permeation, less commonly used today	Zona hardening; increased vacuoles	Prefer EG/DMSO blends; optimize time-concentration exposure[8]

TABLE 3: Vitrification and warming—common errors and stepwise troubleshooting.

Step	*Common errors*	*Corrective action*
Equilibration (E1)	CPA toxicity due to prolonged exposure	Limit to 6–10 minutes; observe shrinkage and re-expansion[7]
Vitrification solution	Delays in plunging into LN_2 → rehydration	Transfer to LN_2 within 1 minute; use precooled straws and pipettes
Warming phase	Inadequate temperature or slow transition	Warm in 37°C sucrose solution; use stepwise dilution (1–3–5–10 minutes) to prevent lysis

(CPA: cryoprotectant agent)

CRYOSTORAGE: INFRASTRUCTURE AND MONITORING

Once vitrified, gametes and embryos must be stored in conditions that ensure their stability for months or years. Mishandling, mislabeling, or environmental hazards such as LN_2 leaks pose risks to both biological safety and legal compliance **(Table 4)**.[10]

REGULATORY AND QUALITY STANDARDS

Compliance with national and international quality control frameworks is vital for sample traceability, patient's protection, and operational excellence **(Table 5)**. Regulatory standards define maximum storage durations, documentation formats, and biobanking principles.

TABLE 4: Cryopreservation safety and infrastructure—common issues and best practices.

Component	*Issue*	*Corrective measures*
Cryotank location	Sunlight exposure, airflow, or vibration leads to temperature shifts	Use a dedicated cryoroom with insulated, epoxy-coated floors (ISO, 2018)
Flooring	Wooden/porous floors → unsafe during LN_2 spill	Use nonslip, nonflammable surfaces like PVC or epoxy resin
Oxygen monitoring	Undetected LN_2 vapor → risk of hypoxia to laboratory personnel	Install realtime oxygen sensors with alarms[8]
Labeling and tracking	Manual errors → misidentification or loss	Implement digital inventory, barcoding, color coding, and double-witness protocols
Documentation	Incomplete cryologs → legal/clinical gaps	Maintain electronic cryologs, fill logs, sample IDs, strict SOPs, and consent-based records[5]
Lack of comprehensive cryopreservation safety measures	Absence of PPE → cryoburns, frostbite, vapor inhalation, injury during transport, or environmental contamination in cryostorage zones	Provide gloves, face shields, cryo-aprons, and tongs for all staff. Use dedicated, appropriately sized trolleys to safely transport cryocans without tipping. Ensure routine cleaning and disinfection of cryo-area surfaces, trolleys, and accessories to maintain sterility and reduce biohazard risk[11]

(ISO: International Organization for Standardization; PPE: personal protective equipment; PVC: polyvinyl chloride; SOPs: standard operating procedures)

TABLE 5: Regulatory and quality standards governing cryopreservation in ART.

Guideline/Standard	*Purpose*	*Application*
ICMR ART Guidelines (India)	National standards for cryopreservation and safety	Define maximum storage durations and identity checks for gametes/embryos
ESHRE (2022)	Best practices in cryopreservation and embryo handling	Benchmarking vitrification and warming steps across accredited ART laboratories
ISO 20387:2018 Biobanking	General biobanking standards for long-term storage	Relevant to institutional donor programs and cross-border gamete shipment

(ART: assisted reproductive technology; ESHRE: European Society of Human Reproduction and Embryology; ICMR: Indian Council of Medical Research; ISO: International Organization for Standardization)

CONCLUSION

Cryopreservation is a delicate intersection of cell biology, chemical precision, and infrastructural integrity. By understanding the nuances of cellular response to cryoinjury, optimizing CPA exposure, and maintaining a tightly regulated lab environment, embryologists can dramatically improve post-thaw survival and clinical outcomes. Compliance with regulatory frameworks like ESHRE and ISO ensures legal and ethical transparency, while investing in staff training and robust documentation prevents errors that could compromise reproductive material. Vigilance at each stage from vitrification to long-term cryostorage is essential for delivering safe, effective, and repeatable results in ART.

REFERENCES

1. Vajta G, Nagy ZP. Are programmable freezers still needed in the embryo laboratory? Review on vitrification. Reprod BioMed Online. 2006;12(6):779-96.
2. De Munck N, Vajta G. Safety and efficiency of vitrification for oocyte and embryo cryopreservation in clinical practice: Considerations for clinical implementation. J Assist Reprod Genetics. 2017;34(11):1533-40.
3. Mazur P. Freezing of living cells: Mechanisms and implications. Am J Physiol Cell Physiol. 1984;247(3):C125-42.
4. Fahy GM. The relevance of cryoprotectant "toxicity" to cryobiology. Cryobiology. 1986;23(1):1-13.
5. Vajta G, Kuwayama M. Improving cryopreservation systems. Theriogenology. 2006;65(1):236-44.
6. Swain JE, Pool TB, Biggers JD. Assessing the quality of culture media for human ART: Current concepts, future prospects. Hum Reprod Update. 2012;18(2):232-47.
7. Kuwayama M, Vajta G, Kato O, Leibo SP. Highly efficient vitrification method for cryopreservation of human oocytes. Reprod BioMed Online. 2005;11(3):300-8.
8. World Health Organization. WHO laboratory manual for the examination and processing of human semen, 6th edition. Geneva: World Health Organization; 2021.
9. ESHRE Guideline Group on Good Practice in IVF Labs. Good practice recommendations for IVF laboratories. ESHRE Guidelines; 2022.
10. International Organization for Standardization. ISO 20387:2018 Biotechnology—Biobanking—General requirements for biobanking. Geneva: ISO; 2018.
11. Van den Bergh M, Bensdorp AJ, van Wely M, Repping S. ICSI versus conventional IVF in patients with non-male factor infertility: A systematic review and meta-analysis. Hum Reprod Update. 2016;22(2):194-200.

CHAPTER

13 Embryo Transfer

INTRODUCTION

Embryo transfer (ET) is the final and arguably one of the most critical steps in the in-vitro fertilization (IVF) process. Despite its apparent simplicity, ET has a significant impact on implantation success and overall, assisted reproductive technology (ART) outcomes. Numerous subtle variables ranging from catheter design and embryo loading protocols to endometrial receptivity and environmental factors can influence implantation rates.[1] The procedure must be executed with a balance of precision, efficiency, and biological understanding to optimize success.

TECHNICAL ASPECTS OF EMBRYO TRANSFER

Transfer Technique

The primary goal during ET is the atraumatic placement of embryos at the optimal location within the endometrial cavity. Transabdominal ultrasound guidance is now considered the standard of care, allowing real-time visualization of catheter placement and embryo deposition and catheter withdrawal.[2] The ideal deposition site is approximately 1.5–2.0 cm below the uterine fundus.[3]

Steps of Ultrasound-guided Embryo Transfer

- The patient is positioned in lithotomy with a moderately full bladder, which helps to straighten the uterocervical angle and enhances endometrial visualization via transabdominal ultrasound.
- A sterile soft ET catheter, usually with an outer sheath, is gently introduced into the cervical canal under continuous ultrasound guidance, minimizing trauma and navigating the path smoothly.
- The catheter is then advanced carefully into the uterine cavity, ideally without touching the fundus, to reduce uterine contractions and avoid trauma.
- Embryos are loaded into the inner sheath in a minimal volume (e.g., 10–20 μL) and are gently deposited in the mid to upper third of the uterine cavity, just below the echogenic endometrial lining and fundal shadow.
- The catheter is withdrawn slowly and steadily to avoid negative pressure, suction, or dragging of the embryo.
- If embryo retention is observed, the catheter should not be flushed or manipulated repeatedly in the operating room. Instead, it should be immediately returned to the incubator under sterile and temperature-stable conditions to preserve embryo viability, and a second attempt should be made only after reloading.
- Minimal personnel should be present in the operating room to reduce air turbulence, distractions, and temperature fluctuations. Avoid repeated door openings during the procedure to maintain thermal and air stability.

- A clean and quiet environment coordinated communication between the clinician and embryologist, and seamless hand-off are critical to optimize outcomes.

Catheter Types and their Selection

Catheters can be broadly categorized into:

- *Soft catheters:* Associated with higher implantation rates due to reduced trauma.
- *Firm catheters:* Easier to insert in difficult cervical anatomy but may provoke contractions.

Selection depends on patient's anatomy and practitioner experience. When difficult transfers are anticipated (e.g., in cases of cervical stenosis), a trial transfer or mock ET should be done in advance to guide catheter choice and technique.

CATHETER PREPARATION AND EMBRYO LOADING

Loading Techniques

Embryo loading should occur in a sterile laminar flow environment using embryo-safe media. Embryos are usually placed between two air bubbles in a minimal volume (10–20 μL) of culture medium.

Common Methods

- *Three-drop method:* Medium–air–embryo–air–medium
- *Air–embryo–air:* Offers precise ultrasound visualization.[4]

Loading must be performed swiftly, ideally within 90 seconds, to minimize embryo exposure to nonoptimal conditions such as ambient temperature fluctuations, pH drift, or osmotic shifts. It is essential to maintain stability in temperature, osmolarity, and pH throughout the ET process. Full flushing of the catheter should be avoided; instead, only the minimal fluid containing the embryos should be released to ensure gentle placement without disturbing the endometrium. During the movement of the loaded catheter from the laboratory to the patient, unnecessary door openings, air drafts, or abrupt physical movements should be avoided, as these can alter the microenvironment and potentially compromise embryo viability and transfer success.

Catheter Warming

Exposure of embryos to nonphysiological temperatures is detrimental. Prewarming the catheter, capillaries, and transfer medium to 37°C avoids cold shock and minimizes uterine contractions.[5] All transfer components should be equilibrated before the procedure.

TIMING OF EMBRYO TRANSFER

The timing of ET must align with the window of implantation (WOI), typically spanning days 19–21 of a regular menstrual cycle. In fresh cycles, ET is coordinated with the rise of progesterone following ovulation. In frozen-thawed embryo transfers (FET), the luteal phase is artificially managed to replicate natural endometrial development.

Blastocyst versus Cleavage Stage Transfers

- *Day 3 (cleavage-stage):* Useful in cases with limited embryo development
- *Day 5 (blastocyst-stage):* Better synchrony with endometrium, higher implantation potential.[6]

Individualization based on patient's history, embryo development, and endometrial receptivity improves outcomes.

ENDOMETRIAL RECEPTIVITY AND WINDOW OF IMPLANTATION SYNCHRONIZATION

Morphological Indicators

- *Endometrial thickness:* 7–14 mm is optimal; <6 mm is associated with poor outcomes.

- *Pattern:* Triple-line (trilaminar) appearance correlates with higher pregnancy rates.
- *Absence of fluid* in the endometrial cavity is essential to prevent embryo displacement.

Biochemical and Molecular Markers

- *Leukemia inhibitory factor (LIF):* A glycoprotein cytokine crucial for embryo-endometrial cross-talk, LIF regulates blastocyst adhesion and invasion by modulating trophoblast differentiation and immune tolerance at the implantation site. Reduced LIF expression is associated with implantation failure, particularly in women with recurrent implantation failure (RIF) and endometriosis.[6]
- *Integrins (αvβ3):* These transmembrane adhesion molecules serve as biomarkers of the endometrial implantation window. αvβ3 integrin expression peaks during the mid-secretory phase and facilitates blastocyst attachment by binding to extracellular matrix ligands like osteopontin. Altered integrin expression is often observed in unexplained infertility.
- *HOXA10 and HOXA11 gene expression:* These homeobox genes regulate endometrial receptivity by controlling stromal cell differentiation and uterine gland development. Their expression is progesterone-dependent and peaks during the implantation window. Dysregulation has been linked to impaired implantation in conditions like polycystic ovarian syndrome (PCOS) and hydrosalpinx.[7]
- *Pinopodes (Uterodomes):* These transient, progesterone-dependent epithelial projections appear on the apical surface of endometrial cells during the receptive phase. Their presence correlates with optimal implantation timing and facilitates close apposition between the embryo and endometrial surface. A lack of pinopodes or asynchronous development is indicative of luteal phase defects or hormonal imbalance.

Endometrial receptivity array (ERA): This molecular diagnostic tool assesses transcriptomic markers in the endometrium to identify the personalized WOI. The ERA testing is especially useful in patients with RIF to guide personalized embryo transfer (pET), ensuring synchronization between embryo development and endometrial receptivity.[8] Recent evidence supports the use of ERA in combination with hormonal replacement therapy or natural cycles, depending on patient's history.

TROUBLESHOOTING COMMON EMBRYO TRANSFER CHALLENGES

Despite being one of the final and seemingly simple steps in the ART process, ET is highly sensitive to minor procedural errors and physiological conditions that can significantly affect implantation and pregnancy outcomes **(Flowchart 1)**. A range of intraprocedural challenges may arise, from technical difficulties in catheter navigation to environmental issues like temperature fluctuations or the presence of endometrial fluid **(Table 1)**. Identifying these potential pitfalls and applying targeted corrective strategies can greatly enhance success rates **(Flowchart 2)**.

INNOVATIONS AND QUALITY STANDARDS IN EMBRYO TRANSFER

- *Catheter design improvements:* Echoenhanced tips and outer sheath guides are in development.
- *Simulation-based training:* ET simulators now help to standardize operator skill.
- *Laboratory-to-clinic coordination protocols:* Real-time communication reduces delays and improves synchronization.

Flowchart 1: Troubleshooting difficult embryo transfer (ET) scenarios.

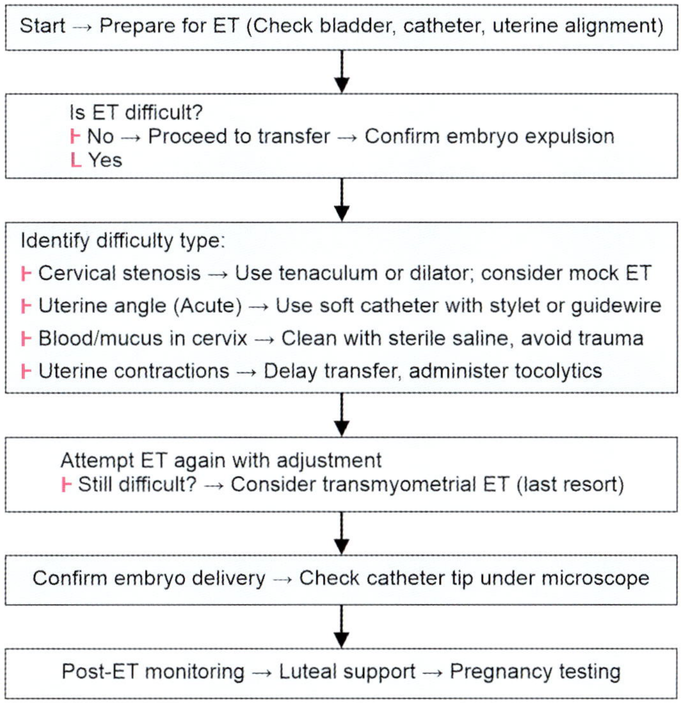

TABLE 1: Troubleshooting common embryo transfer challenges and their impact on ART outcomes.

Issue	*Impact on outcome*	*Corrective strategy*
Difficult cervix	Extended manipulation → trauma, contractions	Use mock transfer; consider using stylet or tenaculum; opt for firm catheter if needed
Uterine contractions	Embryo expulsion, reduced implantation	Avoid touching fundus; perform gentle insertion; use antispasmodics if needed
Bleeding	Contaminated catheter; impaired embryo implantation	Ensure gentle handling; delay transfer or switch to FET if heavy bleeding occurs
Misplaced air bubbles	Wrong embryo location	Practice precise loading technique; confirm under ultrasound before catheter withdrawal
Embryo adherence to catheter	Incomplete deposition	Inspect catheter tip post-transfer; repeat transfer if needed
Cold catheter or medium	Uterine contractions; embryo thermal stress	Prewarm catheter and media; maintain dish on heating stage
Prolonged loading time	Media pH and osmolarity shifts; embryo stress	Limit loading to under 2 minutes; coordinate closely with clinician
Presence of endometrial fluid	Embryo displacement, implantation failure	Cancel fresh transfer and freeze embryos; treat underlying endometritis or progesterone

(ART: assisted reproductive technology; FET: frozen embryo transfer)

Flowchart 2: Step-by-step identification of key factors affecting pregnancy outcome.

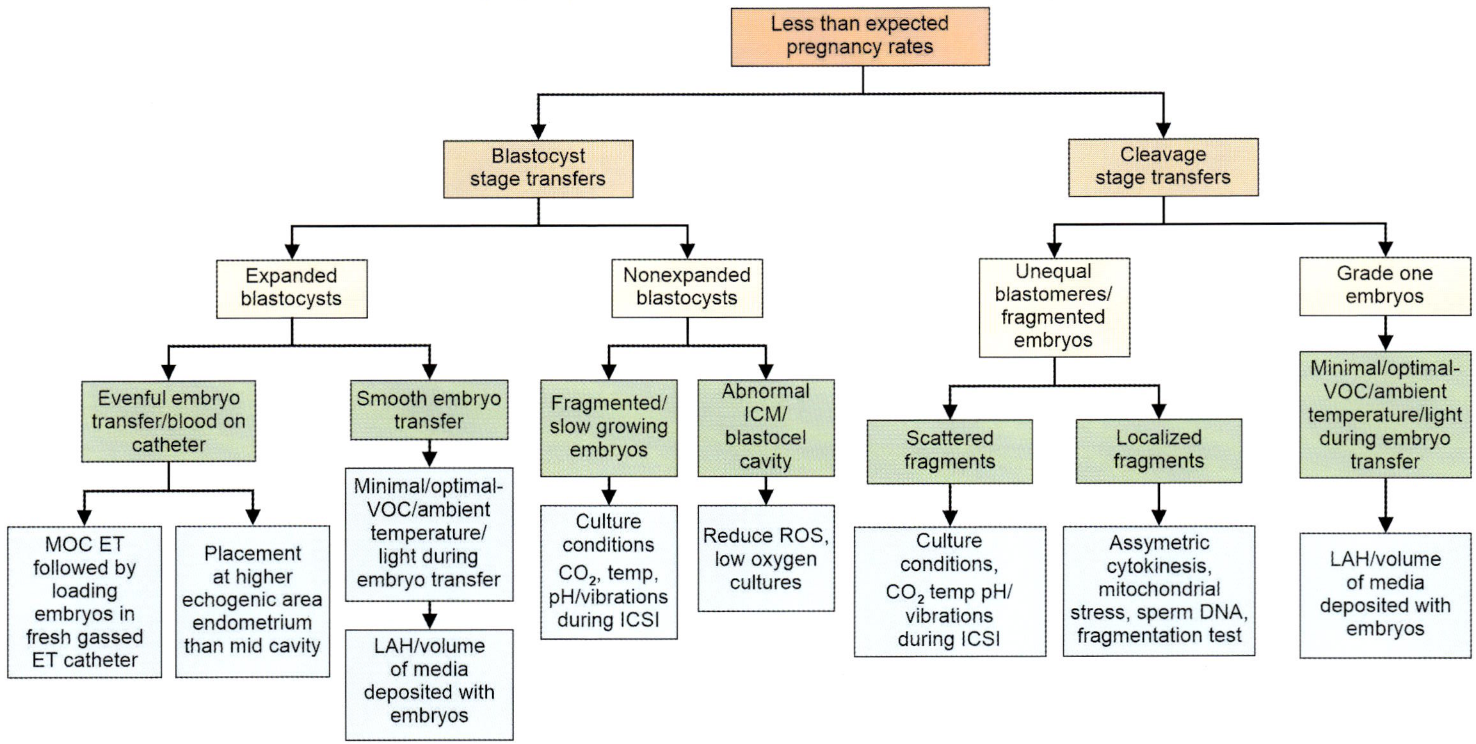

(ET: embryo transfer; ICM: inner cell mass; ICSI: intracytoplasmic sperm injection; LAH: laser-assisted hatching; ROS: reactive oxygen species; VOCs: volatile organic compounds)

CONCLUSION

Embryo transfer is a critical phase in ART, blending technical precision with biological understanding. Although the procedure may appear simple, its success hinges on the seamless coordination of multiple factors—including gentle catheter navigation, optimal embryo loading, accurate placement within the uterine cavity, and the timing of transfer tailored to the endometrium's receptivity. Equally important are patient-specific considerations such as age, hormonal profile, and embryo development stage. Environmental control during transfer, minimizing air currents, limiting uterine irritation, and avoiding unnecessary movements from laboratory to transfer room can further influence outcomes. Innovations such as ultrasound-guided ET, soft-tipped catheters, and molecular assays assessing endometrial receptivity have improved precision, but individualized decision-making remains essential. By integrating internationally accepted protocols with constant refinement through troubleshooting and interdepartmental communication, embryologists and clinicians can significantly improve implantation success and overall ART outcomes.

REFERENCES

1. Schoolcraft WB, Surrey ES, Minjarez DA, Stevens JM, Gardner DK. A prospective randomized trial of uterine contractility and embryo transfer success. Fertility and Sterility. 2001;76(3):418-22.
2. Prapas Y, Prapas N, Hatziparasidou A, Prapa S, Nijs M, Vanderzwalmen P, et al. Atraumatic embryo transfer with a full bladder and transabdominal ultrasound guidance significantly improves pregnancy rates.Fertilility and Sterility. 2019;94(4):1340-4.
3. Woolcott R, Stanger J. Ultrasound tracking of the movement of the air bubble and the embryo post embryo transfer. Hum Reprod. 1997;12(1):137-40.
4. Moreno C, Ruiz A, Simon C, Pellicer A, Remohí J, Serra V. The efficiency of embryo transfer is dependent on the time the embryo spends outside the incubator and on the catheter used. Fertility and Sterility. 2004;82(5):1177-80.
5. Tremellen KP, Valbuena D, Landeras J, Ballesteros A, Martinez J, Simón C. A prospective study examining the impact of pre-warming embryo transfer catheters on pregnancyoutcome. Human Reproduction. 2000;15(9):1872–6.
6. Blake D, Farquhar C, Johnson N, Proctor M. Cleavage stage versus blastocyst stage embryo transfer in assisted conception. Cochrane Database Syst Rev. 2007;(4):CD002118.
7. Mains LM, Van Voorhis BJ. Optimizing the technique of embryo transfer. Fertil Steril. 2010;94(3):785-90.
8. Ruiz-Alonso M, Blesa D, Díaz-Gimeno P, Gómez E, Fernández-Sánchez M, Carranza F, et al. The endometrial receptivity array for diagnosis and personalized embryo transfer as a treatment for patients with repeated implantation failure. Fertil Steril. 2013;100(3):818-24.

SECTION

5 Advanced Manipulations and Ethics

CHAPTER 14

Laser-assisted Hatching and Biopsy Techniques

INTRODUCTION

Advances in micromanipulation techniques have allowed reproductive medicine to push the boundaries of diagnostic and therapeutic intervention, particularly through laser-assisted methods such as laser-assisted hatching (LAH) and embryo biopsy. These techniques have become pivotal tools in embryology laboratories, offering enhanced precision in manipulating the zona pellucida (ZP) and extracting embryonic material for genetic analysis. While LAH primarily supports implantation by facilitating embryo escape from the zona, embryo biopsy allows for genetic assessment via preimplantation genetic testing (PGT).[1] Both procedures, however, require meticulous execution under strict laboratory conditions, as even minor deviations in timing, laser parameters, or handling techniques can cause irreversible damage to embryos, affect hatching potential, or compromise genetic integrity.

SCIENTIFIC BASIS AND INDICATIONS FOR LASER-ASSISTED HATCHING

The ZP is a multiglycoprotein extracellular matrix that encases the mammalian oocyte and preimplantation embryo, playing vital roles in fertilization, protection, compaction, and ultimately, the hatching process. In vivo, the embryo naturally hatches from the zona at the blastocyst stage, typically around day 5–6 of development, to enable trophoblast invasion into the endometrium. In vitro culture conditions, however, may result in zona hardening due to the absence of uterine proteases or due to postcryopreservation changes in zona composition.[2] LAH was thus introduced to mimic this natural process and aid implantation in select patient populations.

Indications for LAH include:

- Advanced maternal age (≥37 years), often associated with reduced embryo quality and increased zona thickness.
- Previous implantation failures despite good-quality embryos
- Embryos with slow cleavage or thickened ZP (>15 μm)
- Cryopreserved and thawed embryos, which exhibit a tendency toward zona calcification or reduced blastocyst expansion.

The timing of LAH is equally critical, with most procedures performed on day 3 cleavage-stage embryos to allow for partial zona thinning, or on day 5 when biopsies or assisted hatching are necessary post-thaw.

LASER SYSTEMS AND TECHNICAL SPECIFICATIONS FOR ZONA MANIPULATION

The most widely used system for laser manipulation in embryology laboratories is the infrared diode laser (typically at a wavelength of 1.48 μm), which is specifically chosen for its ability to be absorbed by water molecules, thus generating highly localized thermal energy with minimal lateral heat dissipation.[3] This property allows for effective zona breaching while preserving adjacent blastomere structures.

Recommended laser parameters:

- *Power:* 100–400 mW depending on the laser model and medium
- *Pulse duration:* 300–500 µs
- *Spot diameter:* 5–7 µm
- *Application:* Multiple pulses spaced apart for thinning; continuous pulses for breaching

Laser manipulation can be classified as either zona thinning, where a linear segment of the zona is attenuated to 30–50% of its original thickness over a 20–30 µm length, or zona opening, where a complete perforation is made (typically 15–20 µm) to facilitate embryo biopsy or immediate hatching.

Excessive laser exposure, particularly when using high-intensity or prolonged pulse durations, can elevate intracellular temperatures or disrupt spindle structures, leading to zona hardening, DNA fragmentation, or delayed development.

TECHNIQUES OF EMBRYO BIOPSY AND THEIR INDICATIONS

Biopsy techniques differ based on the developmental stage of the embryo and the genetic testing intended.

Polar Body Biopsy (Day 0–1)

This method isolates the first and/or second polar body for analysis of maternal genetic contribution. Though minimally invasive, it excludes paternal contributions and is limited in application to monogenic diseases where maternal inheritance is the sole concern.

Cleavage-stage Biopsy (Day 3)

Involves removal of 1–2 blastomeres from a 6–8 cell embryo. Although previously common, it is now discouraged due to high mosaicism rates and the potential to impair embryonic development following the extraction of a large cell fraction.[4]

Trophectoderm Biopsy (Day 5–6)

The most widely accepted approach for PGT, trophectoderm (TE) biopsy involves removing 5–10 cells from the TE, leaving the inner cell mass (ICM) intact. TE biopsy is typically preceded by zona breaching on day 3 to facilitate TE herniation by day 5–6, enabling cell removal with minimal disruption to embryonic polarity or implantation potential.[5]

The biopsy is usually performed using a biopsy pipette (18–22 µm inner diameter), with careful aspiration followed by discrete laser pulses to detach the selected cells. Postbiopsy, embryos are often cultured for 1–3 hours before vitrification to allow re-expansion and structural stabilization.[6]

EQUIPMENT CALIBRATION AND MICROMANIPULATION CONDITIONS

The precision required for both LAH and biopsy mandates strict calibration of micromanipulation systems. The laser system must be tested daily using test slides to confirm beam diameter, focus, and pulse uniformity. Micromanipulators should be aligned to ensure axial accuracy between holding and biopsy pipettes. Holding pipettes are typically 25–30 µm in diameter, while biopsy pipettes should be polished, sterile, and beveled to allow gentle aspiration.

Maintaining the temperature of the micromanipulation stage at 37°C is essential, as even slight deviations can cause ZP contraction, destabilize spindle structures, and impair oocyte viability. The medium used must be properly buffered and equilibrated to a pH of 7.2–7.4 and supplemented with albumin to reduce adhesion of gametes and pipettes to the dish surface. Laser settings used for assisted hatching or biopsy procedures must be accurately calibrated, ensuring consistent pulse energy and targeting to prevent collateral damage to blastomeres or zona.[2] Micropipette bore size must be chosen appropriately based on embryo size and membrane resistance. The precision of the operator in terms of hand stability, axis alignment, and sperm deposition near the polar body significantly influences fertilization success.[7] The micromanipulation equipment should be positioned in a vibration-free, temperature-controlled room with minimal airflow disturbances. Moreover, the injection speed and plunger responsiveness should be finely tuned, especially in hydraulic or pneumatic systems, to ensure a smooth and rapid sperm release with minimal cytoplasmic disturbance.

TROUBLESHOOTING COMMON ISSUES IN LASER-ASSISTED HATCHING AND BIOPSY

Embryos undergoing LAH or biopsy are particularly sensitive due to their developmental stage and structural fragility, and even minor deviations in handling, suction force, or laser settings can significantly impair their ability to re-expand, hatch, or yield viable DNA for analysis **(Flowchart 1)**. It is therefore critical that embryologists follow strict timing, temperature control, and precision-guided movements, along with validated protocols, to prevent damage and enhance the success rates of these delicate ART interventions **(Table 1)**.

Flowchart 1: Biopsy troubleshooting and embryo survival follow-up.

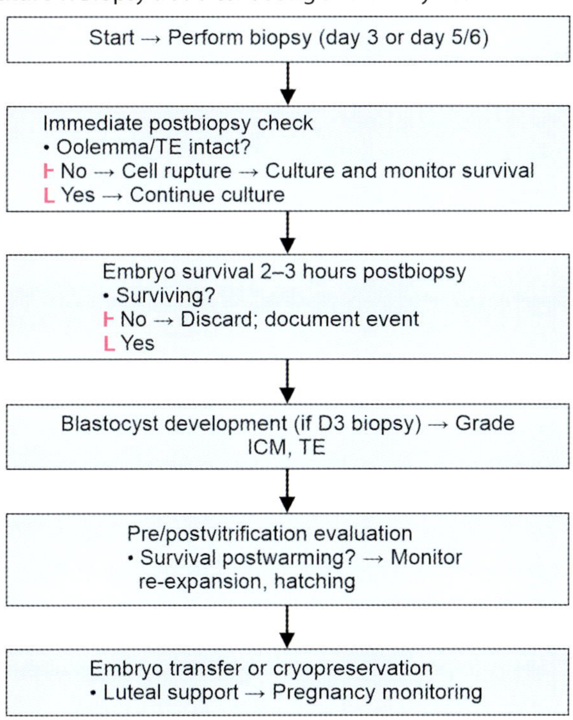

(ICM: inner cell mass; TE: trophectoderm)

TABLE 1: Troubleshooting in embryo biopsy and genetic testing procedures.

Problem	*Likely cause*	*Impact*	*Recommended solution*
Zona hardening post-thaw	Cryopreservation-induced protein crosslinking	Impaired hatching, reduced expansion	Perform partial zona thinning prethaw or postwarming
Blastomere lysis during biopsy	Excess suction and improper pipette angle	Loss of embryo viability or genetic material	Use gentle aspiration, adjust pipette diameter and placement
Embryo collapse postbiopsy	Prolonged manipulation and thermal shock	Impaired re-expansion, developmental arrest	Shorten biopsy duration; culture in prewarmed media
Incomplete zona breach	Low laser energy or poor focus	Delayed TE herniation and difficult biopsy access	Recalibrate laser; increase pulse count if needed
Laser-induced damage	Excessive power or incorrect targeting	Cell lysis and mitochondrial injury	Use lowest effective pulse; avoid direct contact with ICM
DNA degradation postbiopsy	Delay in sample processing or suboptimal lysis buffer	Inconclusive or failed PGT results	Immediately transfer biopsied cells to PCR-compatible buffer

(ICM: inner cell mass; PGT: preimplantation genetic testing; TE: trophectoderm)

ETHICAL AND REGULATORY COMPLIANCE

Biopsy and LAH are governed by strict ethical and legal frameworks to ensure safety, accuracy, and informed consent. European Society of Human Reproduction and Embryology (ESHRE) and Preimplantation Genetic Diagnosis International Society (PGDIS) emphasize the use of standardized protocols, dual witnessing, detailed documentation, and the use of validated media and tools. In India, assisted reproductive technology (ART) clinics must also adhere to the ART Act 2021 and guidelines issued by the Indian Council of Medical Research (ICMR), including maintaining logs of biopsy events, genetic counseling documentation, and sample storage records.

CONCLUSION

Laser-assisted hatching and embryo biopsy represent critical micromanipulation techniques that significantly enhance the diagnostic and clinical success of ART when executed with precision, scientific understanding, and ethical oversight. Mastery of laser calibration, embryo stage-specific handling, zona manipulation strategies, and postbiopsy care is essential to maintain embryo viability while maximizing diagnostic yield. As the field of preimplantation diagnostics continues to evolve, the embryologist's role in applying these techniques responsibly and effectively remains central to the advancement of reproductive medicine.

REFERENCES

1. De Rycke M, Liebaers I, Desmyttere S, Verpoest W, Staessen C, Sermon K, et al. Preimplantation genetic diagnosis and screening: current status and future prospects. Human Reproduction. 2015;30(12):2736-48.
2. Zhao J, Xu B, Zhang Q, Li Y. Effectiveness of laser-assisted hatching on pregnancy outcomes in frozen embryo transfer cycles: A meta-analysis. J Assist Reprod Genetics. 2021;38(3):675-84.
3. Antinori S, Licata E, Dani G, Cerusico F, Versaci C, Antinori M. Zona thinning with laser: impact on fertilization and embryo hatching. Hum Reprod. 2002;17(12):3271-5.
4. ESHRE PGT Consortium. Good practice recommendations for embryo biopsy and handling. Hum Reprod Open. 2020;2020(1):hoz028.

5. Scott RT Jr, Upham KM, Forman EJ, Hong KH, Scott KL, Taylor D, et al. Blastocyst biopsy with comprehensive chromosome screening significantly increases in vitro fertilization implantation and delivery rates. Fertil Steril. 2013;100(3):697-703.
6. Gardner DK, Lane M. Culture and selection of viable blastocysts: a feasible proposition for human IVF? Hum Reprod Update. 2003;9(1):45-56.
7. Kanyo K, Zeke J, Szücs M, Cseh S. Experience with mechanical and laser-assisted hatching. Fertil Steril. 2005;83(6):1513-5.

CHAPTER

15 Consumables and Media Quality

INTRODUCTION

In assisted reproductive technology (ART), the precision of biological procedures relies not only on operator expertise but also critically on the quality, consistency, and handling of laboratory consumables and media. Media used for gamete washing, insemination, embryo culture, vitrification, thawing, and transfer along with plasticware such as pipettes, petri dishes, test tubes, and embryo transfer catheters must meet the highest standards of biocompatibility, sterility, and physicochemical stability. Even minor deviations in storage temperature, exposure to ambient light, or unnoticed expiration can compromise the media's buffering capacity, osmolarity, or protein stability can result in irreversible damage to gametes and embryos.[1]

Ensuring the optimal performance of media and disposables requires rigorous quality control practices, a sound understanding of biological responses to media components, and traceability from procurement to disposal. This chapter outlines common challenges and solutions associated with shelf life, handling errors, lot variability, and traceability in ART laboratories.

SHELF LIFE, EXPIRATION, AND POSTOPENING STABILITY

Every ART consumable and reagent is supplied with a defined shelf life, determined through real-time and accelerated stability studies **(Table 1)**. However, real-world stability also depends on transport conditions, cold-chain integrity, and adherence to postopening usage protocols.

TABLE 1: Troubleshooting issues related to expiry and shelf-life of culture media and plasticware.

Issue	*Scientific impact*	*Corrective measures*
Use of expired media	Breakdown of amino acids, loss of buffering capacity, increased ammonia and reactive oxygen species formation, and decreased embryo viability[2]	Use media within the manufacturer's shelf life. Adopt first expiry first out (FEFO) stock rotation. Never use media even a day past expiry
Extended postopening use	Once opened, media are vulnerable to air contamination, oxidation, and pH drift. Even within expiry, opened bottles degrade faster[1]	Record the date and time of opening. Follow manufacturer guidelines (e.g., use within 7 days postopening with foil resealing). Store under nitrogen or argon overlay when required
Storage of plastics beyond expiry	Degradation of sterilization efficacy, leaching of plasticizers, or compromised packaging sterility	Never stock >3 months' worth of plasticware; inspect sterile packaging integrity visually before use. Avoid exposure to fluctuating temperatures or humidity. Discard expired material immediately to avoid confusion

TABLE 2: Troubleshooting temperature and light-related degradation of IVF media.

Parameter	*Scientific/practical impact*	*Best practices*
Refrigerator malfunction	Prolonged exposure above 8°C or freezing below 0°C leads to irreversible protein denaturation and pH shift	Maintain calibrated digital thermometers and alert systems. Store backup ice packs or use powered medical-grade refrigerators. Have temperature sensor with external display
Media freezing	Crystal formation disrupts matrix structure of proteins; altered osmolarity upon thawing[4]	Never use media that has been accidentally frozen; discard entire lot if suspected freeze exposure
Repeated warming-cooling	Repetitive thermal cycling leads to oxidative stress buildup, reduced amino acid stability, and altered viscosity[5]	Aliquot media in 1–2 mL volumes for one-time use. Warm only what is needed per procedure. Use warmers at 37°C with calibration logs
Light exposure	Photodegradation of riboflavin, folic acid, and other vitamins; ROS formation; pH instability[6]	Wrap bottles in foil. Minimize light exposure of culture dishes. Store in opaque or amber-colored containers

(IVF: in-vitro fertilization; ROS: reactive oxygen species)

STORAGE AND TEMPERATURE STABILITY OF MEDIA

Most ART media contain temperature-sensitive compounds such as bicarbonate buffers, energy substrates (e.g., pyruvate), growth factors, or antibiotics. Deviations from the recommended storage temperature (usually 2–8°C for liquid media) accelerate degradation processes, alter pH, and impair protein activity **(Table 2)**.[3]

LOT-TO-LOT VARIABILITY AND BATCH QUALIFICATION

Despite adherence to Good Manufacturing Practice (GMP) and International Organization for Standardization (ISO) 13485 by media manufacturers, variability persists between production batches, especially for components of biological origin such as human serum albumin (HSA), recombinant proteins, and phenol red **(Flowchart 1)**. These can influence embryo development dynamics, implantation rates, and even methylation patterns of early embryonic genes **(Table 3)**.[6]

Flowchart 1: Lot validation and media batch testing protocol.

Media/lot received → Inspect packaging and label

↓

Check certificate of analysis (COA)
- Sterility, endotoxin, pH, and osmolality

↓

Lot validation setup
- Mouse embryo assay (MEA)
- Sperm survival test

↓

Incubation period
- 24–48 hours for MEA → ≥80% blastocyst formation

↓

Result evaluation
- Pass → Approve lot for clinical use
- Fail → Quarantine lot, report manufacturer

↓

Documentation → Lot release certificate signed

CROSSCONTAMINATION AND PACKAGING ERRORS

Consumables must be certified as endotoxin-free, nontoxic, and embryotoxicity-tested [mouse

TABLE 3: Troubleshooting lot-to-lot variability in ART laboratory consumables.

Lot difference	*Impact*	*Laboratory strategy*
Culture media lot change	Altered blastulation timing, abnormal cleavage patterns, and differing osmolality[3]	Conduct parallel validation using low-quality control embryos or mouse embryo assay (MEA); prequalify with sperm survival test if embryos unavailable
Albumin batch variability	Changes in endotoxin level, hormone contaminants, and lipid content affect zona hardening and embryo compaction	Maintain documentation for albumin lot certificates. Validate with control ICSI runs before routine use
Hyaluronidase lot change	Different enzymatic activity affects oocyte denudation timing, cumulus dispersal, and zona sensitivity	Calibrate exposure time per batch (~30 seconds average). Use test oocytes for batch validation if available
PVP viscosity variation	Influences sperm immobilization and injection speed during ICSI	Confirm pipette drag time with fresh batch; adjust concentration or injection technique accordingly

(ART: assisted reproductive technology; ICSI: intracytoplasmic sperm injection; PVP: polyvinylpyrrolidone)

TABLE 4: Quality hazards in ART media and consumables—impact and mitigation strategies.

Hazard	*Effect on ART outcomes*	*Mitigation strategy*
Microbial/fungal growth in media	Even subclinical bacterial contamination can induce metabolic stress, ammonia buildup, and degeneration	Inspect every media bottle for turbidity or gas formation before use. Use sterility-tested batches
VOC absorption by plasticware	VOCs (e.g., formaldehyde, toluene) from cleaning products or storage rooms can be absorbed by plastics, leaching into culture systems	Use VOC-free cleanroom storage; validate plasticware under controlled room air (CRA) standards
Labeling mismatches	Misidentification of media can result in wrong pH, osmolarity, or HEPES/bicarbonate buffering, risking gamete damage	Barcode scanning, double-witnessing, and segregated storage per media type (HEPES vs. bicarbonate)

(ART: assisted reproductive technology; HEPES: 4-(2-hydroxyethyl)-1-piperazineethanesulfonic acid; VOCs: volatile organic compounds)

embryo assay and limulus amebocyte lysate (MEA and LAL)]. Improper packaging, incorrect storage conditions, or compromised sterility can introduce microbial, particulate, or chemical contaminants that silently impair embryo development **(Table 4)**.[7]

TRACEABILITY, DOCUMENTATION, AND COMPLIANCE

Regulatory frameworks such as the Indian Council of Medical Research (ICMR) ART Guidelines (India), European Society of Human Reproduction and Embryology (ESHRE) laboratory protocols, and ISO 20387 for biobanking emphasize traceability, batch validation, and usage logging.[8] Any deviation from traceable supply chain can lead to legal issues, loss of certification, or unexplainable outcome variation **(Table 5)**.

CONCLUSION

In ART, the invisible errors stemming from consumables and media can be the most

TABLE 5: Quality control documentation in ART laboratories—traceability and compliance tools.

Component	*Role in ART laboratory practice*	*Compliance tools*
Lot and batch traceability	Allows retrospective review of any gamete or embryo loss linked to consumable error	Maintain logs for every consumable/media used in each cycle. Match lot numbers in cryolog, ET sheets, and laboratory reports
Certificates of analysis (COA)	Verifies sterility, endotoxin levels, MEA results, and manufacturer's quality release	Demand COA for every new batch. File in digital inventory with batch name
Inventory and usage logs	Prevents expired or unqualified material usage	Digital logbooks, expiry tracking alarms, and barcode-integrated LIS
Audits and supplier qualification	Ensures vendor compliance with CE-IVD, ISO 13485	Re-audit every 1–2 years or postperformance complaints; document feedback with vendor

(ART: assisted reproductive technology; ET: embryo transfer; LIS: laboratory information system; MEA: mouse embryo assay)

consequential. From temperature-induced protein denaturation and photodegradation of media to lot variability and improper storage conditions, every variable must be controlled and documented with precision. By incorporating rigorous validation protocols, continuous monitoring, and laboratory-wide awareness, embryologists can shield gametes and embryos from unseen threats, safeguarding developmental competence and clinical success. Regulatory adherence, supplier audits, and traceability are not merely bureaucratic measures but foundations of good laboratory practice in reproductive medicine.

REFERENCES

1. Swain JE, Pool TB. ART failure: does it relate to egg, sperm, embryo, or laboratory quality? Fertil Steril. 2008;90(5):1203-8.
2. Bavister BD. Culture of preimplantation embryos: facts and artifacts. Hum Reprod Update. 1995; 1(2):91-148.
3. Van den Abbeel E, Balaban B, Ziebe S, Lundin K, Cuesta MJ, Klein BM, et al. Association between blastocyst morphology and outcome of single-blastocyst transfer. Reprod BioMed Online. 2013;27(4):353-61.
4. Gardner DK, Lane M, Stevens J, Schlenker T, Schoolcraft WB. Blastocyst score affects implantation and pregnancy outcome: towards a single blastocyst transfer. Fertil Steril. 2000; 73(6):1155-8.
5. ESHRE. ESHRE Guidelines for Good Practice in ART Laboratories. Eur Soc Hum Reprod Embryol. 2022.
6. Van Blerkom J, Davis P, Alexander S. Inner mitochondrial membrane potential, cytoplasmic ATP content and free Ca^{2+} levels in metaphase II mouse oocytes. Hum Reprod. 1998;13(6):1469-77.
7. ISO 20387:2018. (2018). Biotechnology—Biobanking—General requirements for biobanking. [online] Available from https://www.iso.org/standard/67888.html [Last accessed December, 2025].
8. ICMR. National Guidelines for ART Clinics in India. Delhi: Indian Council of Medical Research; 2021.

CHAPTER

16 Documentation and Sample Identity

INTRODUCTION

Accurate documentation, sample identity management, and traceability systems are the cornerstones of safe and successful assisted reproductive technology (ART) practice. ART laboratories handle some of the most sensitive biological materials in clinical medicine: gametes, embryos, and cryopreserved specimens which are not only irreplaceable but also subject to strict regulatory and ethical oversight.[1] A single error in labeling, sample tracking, or recordkeeping can lead to devastating consequences such as embryo misplacement, legal action, and loss of patient trust.[2]

The complexity of ART workflows, which often involve multiple steps across different platforms (insemination, fertilization checks, embryo culture, cryostorage, and transfer), demands robust systems for identity verification, procedural documentation, and retrospective audit trails. As laboratories strive to optimize outcomes while adhering to national and international regulations, the integration of quality management systems that emphasize traceability and sample integrity has become indispensable.

IMPORTANCE OF DOCUMENTATION IN ASSISTED REPRODUCTIVE TECHNOLOGY LABORATORIES

Documentation in ART serves several critical purposes **(Table 1)**:

- *Medical and scientific validation:* Clinical records ensure each intervention—intracytoplasmic sperm injection (ICSI), vitrification, and thawing is traceable to outcomes (e.g., fertilization and embryo development).

TABLE 1: Types of documentation in assisted reproductive technology laboratories—purpose and examples.

Type of documentation	*Purpose*	*Examples*
Clinical logs	Record patient's procedures and consent	IVF cycle sheets, and treatment timelines
Laboratory worksheets	Trace sample handling and outcomes	Oocyte retrieval logs and embryo grading forms
Cryostorage logs	Document entry, retrieval, and storage of frozen samples	Dewar fill logs and straw-labeling records
Incident reports	Capture deviations and nonconformities	Broken straw report and thaw-survival failure form
Witnessing logs	Document dual verification of identity-critical steps	Double witnessing forms for insemination and embryo transfer

- *Legal protection and ethical accountability:* Proper documentation protects both the institution and patients in case of disputes or adverse events.
- *Quality assurance:* Accurate logs support internal audits, standard operating procedure (SOP) adherence, and continuous improvement efforts.[3]

Meticulous recordkeeping should be electronic (where feasible), real-time, and secured with restricted access. Backup systems, both digital and paper, must be maintained in line with institutional and legal retention policies. Various witnessing systems are now employed in ART laboratories to ensure sample traceability and procedural accuracy; including infrared (IR) witnessing, barcode-based systems, radiofrequency identification (RFID) tags, and digital double-witness platforms. Each offers advantages such as reduced human error, automatic alerts, and real-time logging, though limitations may include high setup costs, occasional technical glitches, or barcode misreads. Despite automation, manual or electronic double-witnessing remains essential for critical procedures such as gamete handling, embryo transfer, and cryostorage allocation, reinforcing accountability and minimizing mix-up risks.

SAMPLE IDENTITY AND WITNESSING: PREVENTING MISMATCH

Sample mix-ups, though rare, are among the most severe and legally sensitive errors in ART. Critical steps such as insemination, ICSI, embryo transfer, and cryopreservation require dual witnessing. Identity verification must include patient's name, unique identifier (e.g., registration number), and date of birth **(Table 2)**.

The use of electronic witnessing systems such as *RI witness*™ adds an additional layer of error-proofing by providing time-stamped, RFID-tagged logging of all identity-critical steps.[4]

TRACEABILITY: CONNECTING EVERY ACTION TO EVERY OUTCOME

Traceability ensures that every gamete, embryo, and procedure is linked back to the patient and forward to the clinical outcome. It also allows laboratories to trace outcomes back to specific reagents, equipment, staff, or batches **(Table 3)**.

TABLE 2: Critical stages of sample identity risk and preventive measures in assisted reproductive technology (ART) laboratories.

Stage	*Risk of identity error*	*Preventive measures*
Semen sample collection	Labeling mix-up and container swap	Use barcode-labeled containers. Collect identity confirmation at the time of sample handover
Oocyte retrieval and scanning	Dish confusion	Individualized labeled dishes preprepared. Staff crosschecks with retrieval sheet
Intracytoplasmic sperm injection	Wrong sperm to oocyte pairing	Witnessing by a second embryologist. Match dish, oocyte ID, and sperm source
Embryo transfer	Embryo swap and patient's mismatch	Ultrasound room witness confirmation; barcode and ID crossmatch with consent form
Cryopreservation	Straw mislabeling or duplication	Color-coded and heat-stamped straws with unique identifiers. Entry in cryolog with batch, straw, and location

TABLE 3: Comprehensive traceability elements and implementation strategies.

Element	*Traceability scope*	*How to ensure*
Biological material	From retrieval to embryo transfer or discard	Maintain unique patient-specific identifiers across all worksheets and cryostorage units
Media and consumables	Lot number to embryo culture batch	Log media batch number in fertilization and culture sheets
Equipment and personnel	Intracytoplasmic sperm injection (ICSI) performed by whom, on which machine	Digital ICSI logs; micromanipulator ID; and staff initials with timestamps
Cryostorage location	Precise straw and tank position	Cryolog with LN2 tank number, canister, goblet, and straw code
Outcome correlation	Pregnancy to embryo quality and transfer details	Link blastocyst score, culture media, catheter used, and operator to implantation result

TABLE 4: Troubleshooting common documentation and traceability issues.

Issue	*Impact on laboratory or patient safety*	*Solution*
Missing or illegible labels	Risk of sample misidentification or discard	Use waterproof and fade-resistant labels. Perform second-person verification before any manipulation
Unrecorded deviations	Undetected protocol failure and loss of audit trail	Implement deviation logbooks; train staff to report minor issues as well[5]
Data inconsistency (e.g., different DOB on consent vs. worksheet)	Legal conflict and invalidation of informed consent	Mandatory cross-verification of all identifiers across documents before cycle initiation[6]
Manual errors in cryolog	Risk of sample loss or misplacement	Adopt electronic cryolog software with unique identifiers and alerts for duplicates
Lack of linking between laboratory data and clinical outcomes	Missed feedback loop for protocol refinement	Establish centralized electronic database linking embryo data to β-human chorionic gonadotropin results, scans, and outcomes

REGULATORY STANDARDS AND GUIDELINES

Several national and international regulatory frameworks govern documentation and traceability:

- *ICMR guidelines (India):* Mandate 5-year record retention, consent documentation, and cryostorage tracking.
- *ESHRE (2022):* Emphasizes witnessing, traceability, and electronic documentation.
- *HFEA (UK):* Requires all patient-linked materials and procedures to be fully auditable.
- *ISO 20387:2018:* Sets standards for biobanking documentation and sample handling.

Failure to comply with documentation and traceability norms can lead to licensing revocation, legal claims, and irreversible loss of trust **(Table 4)**.

CONCLUSION

Documentation, sample identity, and traceability are not merely administrative aspects of ART practice, they are ethical imperatives and clinical necessities. From patient's safety to legal accountability, the ability to trace every sample, every action, and every result is fundamental to quality reproductive care. With the increasing complexity of ART procedures and rising volumes of cryopreserved material, laboratories must adopt robust digital systems, training protocols, and auditing mechanisms to uphold the highest standards of care. A culture of vigilance, transparency, and accountability can prevent the rare but catastrophic events that compromise both science and human dignity.

REFERENCES

1. ESHRE. Guidelines for Good Practice in IVF Laboratories. Eur Soc Hum Reprod Embryol; 2022.
2. Lutjen P, Trounson A, Leeton J, Findlay J, Wood C, Renou P. The establishment and maintenance of pregnancies using in vitro fertilization and embryo transfer. Fertil Steril. 1984;42(5):753-8.
3. ISO 20387:2018. (2018). Biotechnology—Biobanking—General requirements for biobanking. [online] Available from https://www.iso.org/standard/67888.html [Last accessed December, 2025].
4. Swain JE. Electronic witnessing, double witnessing, and patient safety in ART laboratories. Hum Reprod. 2010;25(11):2675-80.
5. HFEA. Code of Practice. UK: Human Fertilisation and Embryology Authority; 2021.
6. ICMR. National Guidelines for Assisted Reproductive Technology Clinics. Indian Council of Medical Research; 2021.

CHAPTER

17

Ethics, Regulations, and Legal Troubleshooting

INTRODUCTION

The rapid evolution of assisted reproductive technology (ART) has outpaced legislative frameworks in many countries, creating a dynamic intersection between medical innovation, bioethics, and legal governance. As ART procedures such as in-vitro fertilization (IVF), surrogacy, gamete donation, embryo freezing, and preimplantation genetic testing become more prevalent, the need for robust ethical oversight and regulatory compliance becomes ever more critical. Ethical lapses or regulatory breaches can result not only in litigation and professional penalties but also in irreversible psychological harm to patients and reputational damage to clinics.

India, in response to growing ART utilization and associated legal gray areas, enacted two landmark legislations: the Assisted Reproductive Technology (Regulation) Act, 2021 and the Surrogacy (Regulation) Act, 2021. Together, these laws aim to standardize ART practices, protect stakeholders, enforce ethical conduct, and ensure transparency and accountability across ART clinics and banks.

However, navigating these legal frameworks poses significant challenges to clinicians, embryologists, and administrators. This chapter presents a scientific and structured approach to identifying and addressing key legal and ethical troubleshooting areas, including compliance with statutory requirements, protection of donor and surrogate rights, data confidentiality, and informed consent procedures.

REGULATORY LANDSCAPE: THE ASSISTED REPRODUCTIVE TECHNOLOGY AND SURROGACY ACTS

The ART (Regulation) Act, 2021 and the Surrogacy (Regulation) Act, 2021 serve as the primary regulatory frameworks in India for reproductive technologies **(Table 1)**.[1,2]

TROUBLESHOOTING LEGAL AND REGULATORY CHALLENGES IN ASSISTED REPRODUCTIVE TECHNOLOGY (TABLES 2 TO 6)

Clinic Registration and Licensing

Issue: Operating without proper ART board registration or using expired licenses.

Impact: Legal action, patient compensation claims, and clinic closure.

All ART clinics must register under the Central ART Registry and obtain a Unique ART Identification Number (UAID). Regular renewals and display of registration are mandatory. Internal audits every 6–12 months are recommended.

Establish a *Patient Grievance Redressal Committee (PGRC)* within the clinic, aligned with board recommendations, to address complaints transparently and amicably before legal escalation.[6]

TABLE 1: Comparative overview of legal provisions under Assisted Reproductive Technology (ART) Act, 2021 and Surrogacy Act, 2021.

Key provision	*ART Act, 2021*	*Surrogacy Act, 2021*
Governing body	National ART and Surrogacy Board	National ART and Surrogacy Board
Registration requirement	Mandatory for all clinics and banks	Mandatory for all surrogacy clinics
Gamete donation	Anonymous donation permitted; donor registry required	Gamete donation not permitted for surrogacy procedures
Surrogacy type	Not addressed	Only altruistic surrogacy allowed; commercial banned
Record keeping	10-year minimum; must be digital and accessible for audit	25-year retention of records for surrogacy cycles
Offences and penalties	Up to 10 years imprisonment and ₹10 lakh fine for violations	Similar penalties for surrogate exploitation and gamete misuse

TABLE 2: Gamete donation and anonymity.

Troubleshooting point	*Explanation*	*Solution*
Donor anonymity breach	ART Act mandates anonymity: identity cannot be disclosed even to the child (Section 16)	Maintain encrypted donor databases with unique IDs and no name linkage; train staff on confidentiality protocols
Multiple donations by same donor	Maximum one donor per one commissioning couple; usage limited to one couple and three cycles (Rule 12)	Implement a centralized tracking system to prevent reuse across clinics
Donor age or health noncompliance	Donors must be 21–55 (sperm) or 23–35 (oocyte), with genetic screening	Establish SOPs for donor screening, maintain signed medical fitness and consent records

TABLE 3: Surrogacy compliance and misuse prevention.

Risk	*Legal context*	*Recommended measures*
Monetary exchange beyond altruistic compensation	Banned under Surrogacy Act	Maintain receipts only for medical expenses; any financial transactions must be traceable and auditable
Unauthorized surrogate recruitment	Only married women aged 25–35 years with one biological child eligible	Maintain updated surrogate eligibility database, cross-verified with Aadhaar and medical proof
Incomplete or fake consent	All parties must sign notarized consent under board supervision	Use standard board-approved templates and submit to National Registry with timestamped uploads

TABLE 4: Record keeping and data confidentiality.

Problem	*Regulatory mandate*	*Solution*
Poor digital traceability	Clinics must maintain electronic records for at least 10 years (ART Act Section 22)	Use secure, encrypted cloud-based EMR systems with regular backups and audit trails[3]
Lack of patient consent documentation	Informed consent must be obtained at every procedural stage	Introduce digital consent forms with OTP verification or biometric acknowledgment
Failure in donor/embryo tracking	Mislabeling may result in criminal charges	Employ RFID/barcoded witnessing systems for all gamete and embryo handling stages[4]

(ART: assisted reproductive technology; RFID: radiofrequency identification)

TABLE 5: Ethical considerations in ART practice.

Ethical concern	*Explanation*	*Best practice*
Informed decision-making	Patients must be made aware of risks, costs, and chances of success	Use visual aids and multilingual consent materials
Nondiscrimination	ART services must be available irrespective of caste, class, or religion	Clear inclusion/exclusion criteria based only on medical grounds
Gender neutrality and child rights	Sex selection is banned under PCPNDT Act and ART Act[5]	Ensure no sex-disclosing terminology is used in laboratory or patient's communication

(ART: assisted reproductive technology; PCPNDT: Preconception and Prenatal Diagnostic Techniques)

TABLE 6: Managing legal disputes and patient's complaints.

Dispute type	*Origin*	*Mitigation strategy*
Embryo mix-up allegations	Lapses in witnessing and poor labeling	Dual witnessing, digital tracking, and maintaining visual documentation (e.g., annotated photos of embryos at transfer)
Surrogacy exploitation claims	Financial transactions and coercion	Document surrogate counseling, expenses, and welfare board approvals
Failed cycle litigation	Unmet expectations and no informed consent	Provide precycle counseling about success rates, alternative options, and potential complications

INTEGRATION OF LEGAL RISK MANAGEMENT INTO ASSISTED REPRODUCTIVE TECHNOLOGY STANDARD OPERATING PROCEDURES

To create a legally resilient ART practice:

- Incorporate legal checklists into every clinical standard operating procedure (SOP).
- Train embryologists and clinicians in legal documentation.
- Perform mock audits biannually.
- Ensure all contracts (donor, recipient, and surrogate) are reviewed by legal counsel.
- Stay updated with evolving amendments to the ART and Surrogacy Acts.

CONCLUSION

The ethical and legal landscape of ART is as complex as it is necessary. As the science of reproduction advances, it is essential that practices remain rooted in transparency, respect for individual rights, and regulatory discipline.[7] Adhering to the ART and Surrogacy Acts, maintaining detailed records, protecting anonymity, and ensuring informed consent are not only legal obligations but also moral imperatives. A proactive, educated, and compliant approach can shield ART practitioners and patients from avoidable distress while upholding the integrity of the reproductive journey.

REFERENCES

1. Assisted Reproductive Technology (Regulation) Act, 2021 Ministry of Health and Family Welfare, Government of India. (2021). The Assisted Reproductive Technology (Regulation) Act, 2021. New Delhi: Government of India. Available from: https://www.indiacode.nic.in/bitstream/123456789/17031/1/A2021-42.pdf.
2. Surrogacy (Regulation) Act, 2021. Ministry of Health and Family Welfare, Government of India. (2021). The Surrogacy (Regulation) Act, 2021. New Delhi: Government of India. Available from: https://dhr.gov.in/documents/acts-circulars.
3. ESHRE Good Practice/Clinical Recommendations for ART European Society of Human Reproduction and Embryology (ESHRE). (2022). Good practice recommendations for assisted reproductive technology. ESHRE Guidelines Committee. Available from: https://www.eshre.eu/Guidelines-and-Legal.
4. Swain JE. ART lab systems: Errors, prevention, and litigation. Reprod Biomed Online. 2011;23(3):265-75.
5. ICMR National Guidelines for ART Clinics Indian Council of Medical Research (ICMR). (2021). National guidelines for accreditation, supervision and regulation of Assisted Reproductive Technology (ART) clinics in India. New Delhi: ICMR. Available from: https://static1.squarespace.com/static/652ba911757eff001fa8a188/1697360146874/ART_Pdf+icmr.pdf.
6. Banerjee M, Rao KR. Legal and ethical challenges in ART in India. J Fam Med Prim Care. 2022;11(5):1895-902.
7. HFEA Code of Practice Human Fertilisation and Embryology Authority (HFEA). (2020). Code of practice. London: HFEA, United Kingdom. Available from: https://www.hfea.gov.uk/media/3437/code-of-practice-annexes-october-2021.pdf.

Index

Page numbers followed by *f* refer to figure, *fc* refer to flowchart, and *t* refer to table.